T0269371

Integrating Pain Treatment into Your Spine Practice

Steven M. Falowski • Jason E. Pope
Editors

Integrating Pain Treatment into Your Spine Practice

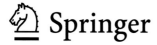 Springer

Editors
Steven M. Falowski, MD
Neurosurgery
St. Luke's University Health Network
Bethlehem, PA, USA

Jason E. Pope, MD, DABPM, FIPP
Summit Pain Alliance
Santa Rosa, CA, USA

ISBN 978-3-319-27794-3   ISBN 978-3-319-27796-7 (eBook)
DOI 10.1007/978-3-319-27796-7

Library of Congress Control Number: 2015959710

Printed on acid-free paper

This Springer imprint is published by Springer Nature
The registered company is Springer International Publishing AG Switzerland

*Nothing would be complete or possible
in my life without the devotion, love, and unwavering
support from my wife, Cindy. Thank you for being my
rock every day and fostering my pursuit of leaving
a mark on our world. Your strength has become my
inspiration, and I look forward to eternity with you.
To my daughter Caroline, who accomplishes
something new each day and makes me smile
endlessly. Daddy will always try to make you proud.
Hard work and dedication does not come easy, for
which I thank you Mom, in showing me through
example the importance and success that it can bring.
To my brother Chris, thank you for keeping my
perspective grounded and thoughts always on family.
My passion and pursuit has always been education.
It is through education that we will change this world
and advance in every regard. To this I must thank my
close friends and fellow workaholics, Jason E. Pope
and David Provenzano, who work by my side in
fostering the same dream.
For all those patients who suffer with chronic pain,
this book is meant to educate and bring awareness to
those physicians who can help.*

Steven M. Falowski, MD

*To my loving children, Liam, Olivia, and Vivienne.
Your joy and awe of the world inspire me to work
towards helping create a better one.
To my wife and partner in all things, Emily. Thank you
for your dedication to our children and your steadfast*

support, grace, and generosity. I am humbled and honored to share this life with you.

To my parents, thank you for your example and advice as I navigate the balance of father, son, husband, and physician.

To Diddi and Poppi for your love and support.

To my twin brother, Greg, thank you for your quiet intellect and demeanor.

To my business partner at Summit Pain Alliance, Dr. Michael Yang. I look forward to the continued success.

To my practice staff at Summit Pain Alliance, thank you for always exceeding my expectations and creating a beacon of hope to help serve the community more completely.

To my friends and colleagues in this pain space, Dr. David Provenzano, Dr. Steven Falowksi, and Dr. Porter McRoberts for their candor, friendship, and support.

To my NANS, ASRA, AAPM, ASIPP, and INS families. Looking forward to many more years of service.

To Timothy Deer, my mentor and friend, thank you for your support, advice, and partnership. We continue to not be victims of circumstance.

Finally, thank you to God, for making all things possible.

Jason E. Pope, MD, DABPM, FIPP

Preface

Spinal surgical intervention is an important treatment tool in the functional and structural restoration of patients. Contrasting one specialty to another, neuromodulation is one that recently has had an unparalleled growth trajectory. This gives a spine surgeon an important role in treating patients throughout their disease process. It is the understanding that a technically successful surgery does not always translate into the patient results that one desires and that the treatment of chronic pain is part of that continuum. Therapies are available when pain persists following surgery, or perhaps when pain is present without a surgical pathology. It is the effort of this book to underscore the concept of concurrent, parallel pathway specialization development, moving away from polarized approaches, towards the integration of pain care in the surgeons' practice. This integration of specialties is the diversity seen in the multidisciplinary approach of the neuromodulation community. The journey has been a rewarding one and we hope to inspire each reader to consider pain care in their practice.

Bethlehem, PA, USA   Steven M. Falowski, MD
Santa Rosa, CA, USA   Jason E. Pope, MD, DABPM, FIPP

Contents

Contributors

Kasra Amirdelfan, MD IPM Medical Group, Inc., Walnut Creek, CA, USA

Jeffrey S. Berger, DO Sports and Spine Rehabilitation Division, Premier Orthopaedic & Sports Medicine, Chadds Ford, PA, USA

Peter G. Campbell, MD Division of Neurosurgery, Parkway Neuroscience and Spine Institute, Hagerstown, MD, USA

Alexios G. Carayannopoulos, DO, MPH Neurosurgery, Comprehensive Spine Center, Brown University Warren Alpert Medical School, Rhode Island Hospital, Providence, RI, USA

Jonathan D. Carlson, MD Interventional Pain, Pain Doctor, LLC, Midwestern Medical School, Glendale, AZ, USA

Ronil V. Chandra, MBBS, MMed, FRANZCR Monash Imaging, Monash Health, Clayton, Melbourne, VIC, Australia

Department of Surgery, Monash University, Melbourne, VIC, Australia

Timothy T. Davis, MD Orthopedic Pain Specialists, Santa Monica, CA, USA

Timothy R. Deer, MD Center for Pain Relief, Inc., Charleston, WV, USA

Steven M. Falowski, MD Neurosurgery, St. Luke's University Health Network, Bethlehem, PA, USA

Daniel A. Fung, MD Orthopedic Pain Specialists, Santa Monica, CA, USA

George M. Ghobrial, MD Department of Neurological Surgery, Thomas Jefferson University Hospital, Philadelphia, PA, USA

Tony Goldschlager, MBBS, PhD, FRACS Department of Surgery, Monash University, Melbourne, VIC, Australia

Department of Neurosurgery, Monash Health, Clayton, Melbourne, VIC, Australia

James S. Harrop, MD Department of Neurological Surgery, Thomas Jefferson University Hospital, Philadelphia, PA, USA

Salim M. Hayek, MD, PhD Department of Anesthesiology, Division of Pain Medicine, Case Western Reserve University, University Hospitals Case Medical Center, Cleveland, OH, USA

Joshua A. Hirsch, MD, FACR, FSIR NeuroInterventional Program, Massachusetts General Hospital, Harvard Medical School, Boston, MA, USA

Bryan C. Hoelzer, MD Anesthesiology and Pain Medicine, Mayo Clinic, Rochester, MN, USA

Chong H. Kim, MD Neurosurgery, Division of Pain Management, Health Sciences Center, West Virginia University, Morgantown, WV, USA

Melinda M. Lawrence, MD Department of Anesthesiology, Division of Pain Medicine, Case Western Reserve University, University Hospitals Case Medical Center, Cleveland, OH, USA

Thabele M. Leslie-Mazwi, MD NeuroInterventional Program, Massachusetts General Hospital, Harvard Medical School, Boston, MA, USA

W. Porter McRoberts, MD Interventional Spine and Pain Medicine, Neurosurgery, Holy Cross Hospital, Fort Lauderdale, FL, USA

Jonathan P. Miller, MD, FAANS, FACS Functional and Restorative Neurosurgery Center, University Hospital Case Medical Center, Cleveland, OH, USA

Neurological Surgery, Case Western Reserve University School of Medicine, Cleveland, OH, USA

Joshua Peloquin, DO Midwestern Medical School, Internal Medicine Intern, Placentia, CA, USA

Julie G. Pilitsis, MD, PhD AMC Neurosurgery Group, Albany Medical College, Albany, NY, USA

Jason E. Pope, MD, DABPM, FIPP Summit Pain Alliance, Santa Rosa, CA, USA

William S. Rosenberg, MD, FAANS Center for the Relief of Pain, Midwest Neuroscience Institute, Kansas City, MO, USA

Joshua M. Rosenow, MD, FAANS, FACS Departments of Neurosurgery, Neurology and Physical Medicine and Rehabilitation, Northwestern University Feinberg School of Medicine, Chicago, IL, USA

Aleka Scoco, BA Case Western Reserve University School of Medicine, Cleveland, OH, USA

Konstantin V. Slavin, MD Department of Neurosurgery, University of Illinois at Chicago, Chicago, IL, USA

Heather C. Smith, BA AMC Neurosurgery Group, Albany Medical College, Albany, NY, USA

Jennifer A. Sweet, MD Functional and Restorative Neurosurgery Center, University Hospital Case Medical Center, Cleveland, OH, USA

Neurological Surgery, Case Western Reserve University School of Medicine, Cleveland, OH, USA

Alexander Vaccaro, MD, PhD Department of Orthopedic Surgery, The Rothman Institute, Philadelphia, PA, USA

Dali Yin, MD, PhD Functional Neurosurgery, University of Illinois at Chicago, Chicago, IL, USA

Youngwon Youn, BA AMC Neurosurgery Group, Albany Medical College, Albany, NY, USA

Part I
Identification and Management of Pain Patients

Chapter 1
Identification of the Pain Patient

Alexios G. Carayannopoulos

Key Points

- It is well established that chronic pain is undertreated and that earlier multidisciplinary pain management intervention may lead to better clinical outcomes.
- Appropriate initial clinical triage should be followed by ongoing clinical reassessment, which should be coordinated across the medical, interventional, and surgical domains. This fosters communication between patients and providers, to ensure that patients are maintaining satisfactory gains in meeting their goals.
- Clinical practice guidelines are essential tools to help guide the treatment of pain patients.
- Because psychological disorders and social influences affect outcomes of patients with chronic low pain, psychological screening and identification of social influences are very important to understand in treating the pain patient.
- A high prevalence of failed back surgery syndrome approaching 40 % suggests that a multidisciplinary approach may be needed to triage candidates appropriately to targeted surgical and nonsurgical pain treatments.

A.G. Carayannopoulos, D.O., M.P.H. (✉)
Neurosurgery, Comprehensive Spine Center, Brown University Warren Alpert Medical
School, Rhode Island Hospital, Providence, RI 02903, USA
e-mail: acarayannopoulos@lifespan.org

© Springer International Publishing Switzerland 2016   3
S.M. Falowski, J.E. Pope (eds.), *Integrating Pain Treatment into Your Spine
Practice*, DOI 10.1007/978-3-319-27796-7_1

Introduction

Spine cases are some of the most common surgeries performed by neurosurgeons and orthopedic surgeons in the USA. Based on the literature, 40 % of patients will suffer from chronic pain following a spinal surgery. It is well established that chronic pain is undertreated and that earlier pain management intervention may lead to better clinical outcomes. Paradoxically, many spine surgeons are unaware of the extent of pain therapies available outside of surgery, nor how to engage patients in a multimodal, multidisciplinary, comprehensive, combined surgical and nonsurgical treatment paradigm. As one of this book's goals is to educate spine surgeons on comprehensive care, the first chapter of this book focuses on "identification of the pain patient," which is the first essential step in successfully engaging the spine patient into this treatment paradigm. Identification of the pain patient requires recognition of a patient suffering from spine-related pain early on. Because spine pain is often accompanied by loss of function and quality of life, earlier recognition and intervention will not only lead to a better clinical outcome but may also prevent disability.

Identification of the pain patient can be done through a multitude of approaches, some of which have been validated through clinical studies, others of which are more anecdotal and have been passed down through generations of spine care, based upon collective years of experience. From the provider's perspective, the goal is to identify patients with spine pain, make an appropriate diagnosis, and then triage the patient into the most appropriate treatment. From the patient's perspective, the goal is to provide the patient with an opportunity to share in the decision-making process with his/her provider in order to achieve the best outcome based upon individualized functional goals. Generally, commonalities of both perspectives include decreased pain, increased function, and enhanced level of satisfaction. Ultimately, working towards these goals together will lead to the best clinical outcome.

Initial Evaluation

The first step in identifying the pain patient begins with clinical triage. Generally, triage is best facilitated by direct communication between two providers. Ideally, clinical triage should route patients to the appropriate surgical or nonsurgical provider and begins with initial assessment of symptoms, general review of treatment objectives, and early identification of red flags to best direct care. In the spine world, red flags include signs or symptoms of progressive motor or sensory neurological deficit, bowel/bladder dysfunction, or extreme pain, which is recalcitrant to conservative measures. Thankfully, the majority of spine cases are nonsurgical and can be successfully managed by medical or interventional options. Only patients who are candidates for and who are interested in pursuing surgery should be triaged to a surgical provider.

For continued identification of the pain patient, an appropriate in-person evaluation must then ensue. All initial evaluations begin with a thorough history, which includes a review of subjective and objective levels of pain and function, review of diagnostic studies, previous interventions, and previous responses to treatment. This is followed by a focused physical examination. Only after careful correlation of subjective and objective findings should attempts be made at an overall assessment, which includes a clinical diagnosis as well as a functional status. Finally a treatment plan, including education, and need for medical, interventional, or surgical options, is created based upon a patient's individualized treatment objectives.

Although patients' goals are often unique, most goals imply a reduction of pain to facilitate an increase in function. Continued clinical reassessment, which is coordinated across the medical, interventional, and surgical domains by a robust triage system, allows ongoing communication between patients and providers to ensure that patients are maintaining satisfactory gains in meeting their goals.

Use of Outcome Measures

Because the treatment of spine-related pain is challenging, in part due to the subjectivity of pain, early use of standardized outcome assessment tools is essential in identifying the pain patient. Assessment tools should include both subjective measurements of pain and psychological distress, as well as objective measurements of function. Baseline testing establishes a reference point, from which patients' pain and function levels are monitored longitudinally. Graphical displays outlining trends can be used to educate, encourage, and reassure patients. Additionally, these data points are helpful to validate progress for insurance companies, as they highlight progression through the treatment paradigm.

There are a number of outcome tools that reflect different domains important in spine care, which can be used to identify the pain patient. These measures assess pain, physical/psychosocial function, and quality of life (see Table 1.1). Furthermore, they can be subdivided into objective measures and preference-based measures

Table 1.1 Assessment tools

Pain	Numeric Pain Rating Scale (NPRS)
	Brief Pain Inventory (BPI)
	Pain Disability Index (PDI)
	McGill Pain Questionnaire
	Visual Analogue Scale (VAS)
Physical function	Owestry Disability Index (ODI)
	Roland Morris Disability Index
	Range of motion (ROM)
Psychosocial function	Fear Avoidance Beliefs Questionnaire
	Tampa Scale for Kinesiophobia
	Beck Depression Inventory (BDI)
Quality of life	Short Form 36 (SF36)
	Nottingham Health Profile (NHP)
	Short Form 12 (SF12)
	Sickness Impact Profile (SIP)

Table 1.2 Subdivided tools

Objective based	• Work status/return to work • Complications or adverse events • Medications used
Preference based	• European Quality of Life (EQ5D) • Short Form 6 (SF6)

(see Table 1.2) [1]. The choice of outcome measure can be daunting. Of the different domains generally assessed, it is felt that pain, function, and quality of life are the most important for identification of the pain patient in both the clinical and research setting. If cost utilization is important, preference-based measures should be used over objective measures.

In summary, for identification of the pain patient, it has consistently been recommended to use both VAS and NRPS secondary to responsiveness and ease of use. For assessment of function, the ODI and RMDQ are recommended. For quality of life, the SF36 and its shorter versions should be used. If cost is important, the EQ5D or SF6 should be used. Psychosocial tools should be used as screening tools prior to surgery because of their inherent lack of responsiveness. Complications should be assessed as a standard of clinical practice. Return to work and medication are not recommended unless these specific questions are being asked. Finally, in deciding on which measures to use, it is suggested that burden in administration to both staff and patients be considered [1].

Multidisciplinary Care

After careful assessment and development of a treatment plan, identified pain patients should be engaged into a multimodal, multidisciplinary treatment paradigm. Historically, the origin of the multidisciplinary approach in the treatment of pain is the legacy of John Bonica, MD, an anesthesiologist and one of the pioneers of pain medicine. Today, the multidisciplinary approach prevails. In fact, use of an independent multidisciplinary assessment for treatment planning, including extensive intake evaluation by a team of therapists, counselors, and a physician, with subsequent generation of a comprehensive report, has been studied and found to provide a potentially reproducible standard for both research and clinical use [2].

Multidisciplinary care includes a continuum of medication management, rehabilitation (physical, occupational, vocational), interventional treatments, psychological co-management, complementary and alternative options, and of course surgical management of pain. After appropriate triage, evaluation, and assessment, placement of the identified pain patient into the appropriate treatment algorithm is guided by a number of tools, as well as their previous treatment history within the multidisciplinary approach.

Clinical Practice Guidelines

Clinical practice guidelines are another essential tool to guide treatment of the identified pain patient. These guidelines present statements of best practice, which are based upon careful and exhaustive assessment of the available evidence from published studies on the outcomes of different treatment options. In November 1989, Congress mandated the creation of the Agency for Healthcare Policy and Research (AHCPR). This organization was given broad responsibility to support research, data development, and related activities. In conjunction with this mandate, the National Academy of Sciences published a document indicating that guidelines were expected to improve the quality, appropriateness, and effectiveness of health care services.

Of the different societies promulgating guidelines, some are more medical, some more interventional, and others more surgical. Examples of each include the American Pain Society (APS) in conjunction with the American College of Physicians (ACP), the American Society of Interventional Pain Physicians (ASIPP), and the North American Spine Society (NASS), respectively. As various society recommendations reflect upon variable vested interests, education, through the use of shared decision, is essential to navigate the various guidelines. Shared decision making helps the patient to negotiate through the different medical, interventional, and surgical treatment options to make an autonomous and informed decision best individualized to meet his/her personal functional goals.

One specific set of medical guidelines by the APS/ACP stands out among these classification systems, which is summarized in the following bulleted recommendations:

- Recommendation 1: Clinicians should conduct a focused history and physical examination to place patients with low back pain into one of the three broad categories including nonspecific low back pain, back pain associated with spinal stenosis or radiculopathy, or back pain associated with another specific spinal etiology.
- Recommendation 2: Clinicians should not routinely obtain imaging or diagnostic studies in patients with nonspecific low back pain.
- Recommendation 3: Clinicians should routinely perform diagnostic imaging and testing for patients with low back pain when severe or progressive neurologic deficits are present or when serious underlying conditions are suspected on the basis of history and physical examination.
- Recommendation 4: Clinicians should evaluate patients with persistent low back pain and signs or symptoms of radiculopathy or spinal stenosis, only if they are potential candidates for surgery or interventional spine treatments.
- Recommendation 5: Clinicians should provide patients with evidence-based information on low back pain with regard to their expected clinical course, advise patients to remain active, and provide self-care options.
- Recommendation 6: For patients with low back pain, clinicians should consider the use of medications, which have proven benefits, in conjunction with back care information and self-care.

- Recommendation 7: For patients who do not improve with self-care options, clinicians should consider the addition of non-pharmacologic therapy, which has proven benefits for acute low back pain, including spinal manipulation. For chronic or subacute low back pain, clinicians should consider including intensive interdisciplinary rehabilitation, exercise therapy, acupuncture, massage therapy, spinal manipulation, yoga, cognitive-behavioral therapy, or progressive relaxation [3].

Because there are a number of clinical practice guidelines for low back pain, which have been characterized by inconsistencies and multiple conflicts in terminology and technique leading to significant diversity in their approach, it is sometimes difficult to implement and adhere to any single guideline consistently [4, 5]. Furthermore, although evidence-based guidelines for evaluation and treatment of chronic low back pain have revealed consistent recommendations and guidance for the *evaluation* of low back pain, unfortunately, there are inconsistent recommendations and guidance for the *treatment* of low back pain. Overall, it is essential to emphasize that clinical guidelines do not represent a "standard of care."

Evidence-based medicine emphasizes the need for rigorous critical appraisals of the scientific literature to inform medical decision making and places strong emphasis on the requirement for valid studies, particularly randomized controlled trials to appropriately evaluate the effectiveness of health care interventions. There is widespread evidence that following evidence-based practice, including clinical practice guidelines, will improve patient outcomes with low back pain and will reduce anecdotal variations in care [6].

Psychosocial Stratification

Because psychological disorders and social influences affect outcomes of patients with chronic low pain, psychological screening and identification of social influences are very important to assess. Understanding of these domains can guide placement of the identified pain patient into appropriate treatment. For example, patients with higher scores on depression and neuroticism scales generally respond more favorably to conservative management over surgery, although the evidence is weak [7]. Likewise, patients with degenerative disc disease (DDD) and a personality disorder respond more favorably to conservative management over patients with DDD without a personality disorder, who respond more favorably to fusion.

Sociodemographic factors should be considered when identifying pain patients and making treatment decisions. Important risk factors include smoking, social support, education level, and job satisfaction. Although these factors alone do not preclude specific treatments, they should be taken into consideration when implementing treatment [8]. Overall, use of a validated psychological screening tool can be helpful in stratifying the identified pain patient, although the evidence is weak.

Procedure-Specific Identification

There are general and treatment-specific clinical practice guidelines for the treatment of chronic non-radicular low back pain. In part, this has arisen because the treatment of DDD with lumbar arthrodesis has risen fourfold in the last several decades. This has led to rise in health care costs, which in turn have increased the prevalence of clinical and payer guidelines, which have had a direct influence on patient and provider treatment options. The availability of evidence-based practices frequently dictates patients' care, often above the autonomous decision of the surgical provider. Because of concerns over efficacy and the direct and indirect costs of surgical treatment with low back pain, surgical spinal fusion in particular has come under increased scrutiny [9].

Several studies have sought to look at efficacy of spinal fusion versus efficacy of conservative treatment measures. It is unclear from the literature which patients with chronic low back pain without neurological impairment are the best candidates for fusion versus conservative management. However, it has been shown that nonsmokers are more likely to have a favorable surgical outcome, while patients with medical comorbidities have a less favorable outcome. Additionally, it has been well established that the success of patients who have had previous spinal surgery having success with repeated spinal surgeries is marginal, at best. Furthermore, interventional spine therapies can achieve higher success rates in the subclass of patients with failed back surgery syndrome (FBSS), with class 1 evidence now demonstrating that spinal cord stimulation is significantly more successful than repeated operations, by multiple outcome measures, in carefully screened and selected patients with FBSS [10]. In fact, SCS was both less expensive than re-operation and economically denominate in terms of cost-effectiveness and cost utility [11].

Summary

Identification of the pain patient is the first step in comprehensive spine care. This is initiated through clinical triage and is continued throughout the multidisciplinary treatment paradigm. Appropriate medical, interventional, and surgical assessment should be balanced with the use of standardized outcome tools to assess baseline levels of pain and function, which are monitored throughout treatment. The identified pain patient is placed into an appropriate treatment plan taking into account their position in the algorithm, which is primarily guided by clinical practice guidelines and secondarily by consideration of psychosocial variables and specific treatment concerns.

Although tremendous variabilities exist in the identification of the pain patient, it has become evident that use of a multidisciplinary approach prevents sliding into the "one-size-fits-all" paradigm commonly seen in the tool bag of medical providers. Surgeons and medical/interventional pain physicians can work in tandem to identify patients in pain early on, to be able to consistently offer therapeutic options that span multiple specialties. Physician awareness is key, and education is paramount.

References

1. Chapman JR, Norvell DC, Hermsmeyer JT, Bransford RJ, DeVine J, McGirt MJ, Lee MJ. Evaluating common outcomes for measuring treatment success for chronic low back pain. Spine. 2011;36 Suppl 21:S54–68.
2. Haig AJ, Geisser ME, Michel B, Theisen-Goodvich M, Yamakawa K, Lamphiear R, Legatski K, Smith C, Sacksteder J. The Spine Team Assessment for chronic back pain disability. Part 1: basic protocol and performance in 500 patients. Disabil Rehabil. 2006;28(17):1071–8.
3. Chou R, Qaseem A, Snow V, Casey D, Cross Jr JT, Shekelle P, Owens DK, Clinical Efficacy Assessment Subcommittee of the American College of Physicians, American College of Physicians, American Pain Society Low Back Pain Guidelines Panel. Diagnosis and treatment of low back pain: a joint clinical practice guideline from the American College of Physicians and the American Pain Society. Ann Intern Med. 2007;147(7):478–91.
4. Manchikanti L, Singh V, Helm II S, Schultz DM, Datta S, Hirsch JA, American Society of Interventional Pain Physicians. An introduction to an evidence-based approach to interventional techniques in the management of chronic spinal pain. Pain Physician. 2009;12(4):E1–33.
5. Ostelo R, Croft P, van der Weijden T, van Tulder M. Challenges in using evidence to inform your clinical practice in low back pain. Best Pract Res Clin Rheumatol. 2010;24(2):281–9.
6. Chou R. Evidence-based medicine and the challenge of low back pain: where are we now? Pain Pract. 2005;5(3):153–78.
7. Daubs MD, Norvell DC, McGuire R, Molinari R, Hermsmeyer JT, Fourney DR, Wolinsky JP, Brodke D. Fusion versus nonoperative care for chronic low back pain: do psychological factors affect outcomes? Spine. 2011;36 Suppl 21:S96–109.
8. Mroz TE, Norvell DC, Ecker E, Gruenberg M, Dailey A, Brodke DS. Fusion versus nonoperative management for chronic low back pain: do sociodemographic factors affect outcome? Spine. 2011;36 Suppl 21:S75–86.
9. Cheng JS, Lee MJ, Massicotte E, Ashman B, Gruenberg M, Pilcher LE, Skelly AC. Clinical guidelines and payer policies on fusion for the treatment of chronic low back pain. Spine. 2011;36 Suppl 21:S144–63.
10. North RB, Kidd DH, Farrokhi F, Piantadosi SA. Spinal cord stimulation versus repeated lumbosacral spine surgery for chronic pain: a randomized, controlled trial. Neurosurg. 2005;56(1):98–106.
11. North RB, et al. Spinal cord stimulation versus reoperation for failed back surgery syndrome: a cost effectiveness and cost utility analysis based on a randomized, controlled trial. Neurosurg. 2007;61:361–9.

Chapter 2
Role of Spinal Surgery in Pain Management

George M. Ghobrial, Alexander Vaccaro, and James S. Harrop

Key Points

- The most common pathologies addressed with spinal surgery are compressive in etiology, and the goal of surgery is decompression of the neural elements.
- Neuropathic pain is complex, often encountered with dysesthetic pain and allodynia. This is indicative of pathology of the central or peripheral nervous tissue, or both.
- While radicular and claudicant-type symptoms are most often associated with compressive lesions of a peripheral nerve, the origin of axial back pain can be multifactorial, which necessitates appropriate work-up.
- Spinal decompression and stabilization are unlikely to adequately relieve neuropathic pain symptoms.
- A high prevalence of failed back surgery syndrome approaching 40 % suggests that a multidisciplinary approach may be needed to triage candidates appropriately to targeted surgical and nonsurgical pain treatments.

G.M. Ghobrial, M.D.
Department of Neurological Surgery, Thomas Jefferson University Hospital,
909 Walnut Street, 3rd Floor, Philadelphia, PA 19107, USA
e-mail: georgeghobrial@gmail.com

A. Vaccaro, M.D., Ph.D.
Department of Orthopedic Surgery, The Rothman Institute,
Philadelphia, PA 19107, USA

J.S. Harrop, M.D. (✉)
Department of Neurological Surgery, Thomas Jefferson University Hospital,
909 Walnut Street, 2nd Floor, COB Bldg., Philadelphia, PA 19107, USA
e-mail: james.harrop@jefferson.edu

© Springer International Publishing Switzerland 2016
S.M. Falowski, J.E. Pope (eds.), *Integrating Pain Treatment into Your Spine Practice*, DOI 10.1007/978-3-319-27796-7_2

Introduction

Back pain due to spinal etiologies accounts for the second most common reason for a patient consultation in the primary care setting [1]. Furthermore, while most back pain is transient, and the time course is self-limiting, the estimated lifetime prevalence of low back pain (LBP) is estimated to be greater than 90 %, which means that nearly all patients will suffer from this ailment at some point in their lives leading to medical consultation [2]. The prevalence and incidence of chronic back pain are even less well understood, in part due to the lack of agreement on the minimum duration of pain that is required in order to meet the definition of chronic pain—often in as few as 7 weeks. The most general definition of chronic pain is where the pain persists beyond the expected time period for a given pathology.

For most patients, symptoms subside after the first-time onset. For the less fortunate, LBP persists after a trial of analgesic medication, and physical therapy, leading to consultation with a spine specialist. Further complicating spinal pain is the large number of patients thought to seek treatment for chronic LBP due to psychiatric, work-related/socioeconomic, or any kind of secondary gain issue [1]. Regardless of the stated reason, longitudinal studies link chronic spinal pain with depression and disability [2, 3]. Obtaining a proper diagnosis of spinal pain is difficult, and requires a careful history from the patient.

As highlighted in Chap. 1, "Identification of Pain Patients," the efficient design of the neurologic or orthopedic surgery practice in patient selection is to maximize appropriate candidates for surgical treatment. Often, those that are given an appointment with a spine surgeon have undergone evaluation by a primary care doctor or clinician with painful symptomatology and have obtained diagnostic imaging suggestive of a corresponding compressive lesion. The authors will highlight in this chapter that not all of these patients may require surgical decompression for neural compromise. Evidence of the complexity of pain generators that are initially overlooked and do not respond to surgical decompression alone is illustrated by the high prevalence of failed back syndrome (FBSS).

As a result, appropriate triage in the spinal practice is needed to ensure that patients with chronic pain without neural element compression may need one or more less invasive alternative interventional and nonsurgical techniques that will be outlined later in this chapter and in more detail in subsequent chapters.

Identification

The most basic definition of FBSS has been the persistence of LBP following spinal surgery [4]. An argument can be made that the higher the percentage of FBSS in a particular clinic, the more the surgeons should be asking themselves if they have appropriately identified candidates for decompressive surgery or adequately exhausted interventional pain management options prior to surgery. Further confounding the issue is the dynamic nature of overstimulation of preoperative nociceptive pathways that may result in a shift of pain generators from the acute pathology to chronic pain. This too can lead to an elevated rate of FBSS.

Nonoperative Measures

A complete in-depth discussion of the various nonsurgical treatment modalities can be found in the subsequent chapters of this book. Overall, the predictors of success for nonsurgical therapies for LBP are not well understood [5, 6]. This is not surprising for many reasons. In the literature, there is a paucity of placebo-controlled randomized studies. When analyzing the prospective studies, the most obvious difficulty in generalization across studies is the lack of standardization of selection criteria, definitions of pain, and validated objective outcome measures for pain. The criteria for diagnosis and inclusion in most studies for facet and epidural injection differ, as well as the criteria for success ranging from 50 % or greater. Chapters 12, 13, and 14 will discuss in more detail the specifics of interventional, neuromodulation, and intrathecal drug therapies available for the nonsurgical treatment of LBP, respectively. However, the authors will highlight below some key points regarding patient selection and nonsurgical treatment of LBP below.

Facet Blocks

One common contributor to axial back pain LBP is facet arthropathy. The facet joints are richly innervated by a dual innervation of somatic, nociceptive, and autonomic pain fibers. Therefore, somatic fibers at each facet level are responsible for characteristically localized pain in tandem with referred pain due to a convergence of pathways with autonomic fibers either in the dorsal horns or thalamus in the second- or third-order ascending pathways, respectively [7]. It is important to consider facet arthropathy as a source of pain, particularly in the setting of axial LBP, without radicular symptoms. The diagnosis of facet joint pain is typically made by an interventional facet nerve block yielding symptomatic relief of LBP in the absence of radiculopathy [8]. Facet pain has been shown in studies by Manchikanti and colleagues to have a prevalence ranging from 20 to 40 % of all LBP [8–15]. There are no class A recommendations for the management of "facet-joint"-type pain. Instead, level II evidence supporting lumbar facet joint nerve blocks [8, 16, 17] and radiofrequency neurotomy [18, 19] has been previously published supporting these modalities of pain mediation. Furthermore, only level III evidence exists in support of intraarticular corticosteroid injections for chronic LBP thought to be due to facet arthropathy [20, 21]. Long-term benefit has been noted with the injection of anesthetics and most recently in 2014 the addition of cortico-steroids yielded no added long-term pain relief beyond that provided by local anes-thetics [8]. Overall, when facet joint pain is overlooked as an etiology of axial LBP, painful symptoms can persist after surgical decompression.

Discogenic Pain

Internal disc disruption (IDD) resulting in discogenic pain is thought to be the most common cause of axial LBP [7]. IDD is defined as degeneration of the disc, desic-cation, and disc height collapse, with annular tears in the absence of disc herniation and neural compression [22]. In the absence of radicular symptoms, an associated herniated disc is rarely thought to be the cause of axial pain. The characteristics of discogenic pain are often ill defined and the relative benefits of open spinal surgery are not as clear compared to interventional or rehabilitative measures. In a systematic review comparing five RCTs, no significant difference in ODI was found between spinal fusion and nonsurgical management [23]. In a long-term follow-up of three RCTs by Mannion and colleagues, no significant difference was seen between the surgical and nonsurgical groups as well [24]. One flaw in these studies is the lack of concordance between choice of nonsurgical therapy and specific surgical interven-tion. Overall, discogenic pain remains as the most common cause of back pain and a uniform surgical approach may not be the answer for each patient. Appropriate localization of the pain generator in the case of multilevel degenerative disc disease is often required.

Evidence

Spinal surgery is justified for a wide number of specific indications pertaining to pain due to neural compromise due to degenerative, oncologic, infectious, vascular, and traumatic indications and is beyond the scope of this chapter. Most of these indications present acutely with spinal pain, due to compression of the neural elements. As such, decompression of the neural elements through direct or indirect means as well as stabilization of the unstable spine are the mechanisms by which acute pain relief is given to the patient. Chronic stimulation of the peripheral nerve receptors by a noxious stimulus can lead the neurons to a state of hyperexcitability, and even lead to spontaneous firing [7]. This condition can lead to a state of hyper-algesia and allodynia not amenable to decompressive spinal surgery, even in the setting of a compressive lesion.

Failed Back Surgery Syndrome

As previously mentioned, up to 40 % of patients undergoing lumbar decompressive surgery with or without fusion do not obtain relief of painful lumbar leg and back symptoms [25]. As a result, patients often undergo evaluation for spinal cord stimulation (SCS) in the office, followed by a trial stimulation period using a less invasive percutaneous electrode stimulation system. With careful patient selection including a trial placement and often psychological screening, up to three-quarters of patients obtain symptomatic relief of chronic leg and back pain seen with a decrease in analgesic medication use and improvement in objective outcome measures of pain and quality of life [25]. One common complaint of SCS is the persistence of limb paresthesias as a result of high-frequency stimulation of the dorsal columns [7]. Technology with SCS is improving further, with a prospective randomized study comparing high-frequency (500 Hz) stimulation, burst stimulation, and placebo finding significant reduction in paresthesias with burst stimulation mode as well as improvement in painful lower extremity symptoms [26].

Most importantly, the successful use of SCS or any spinal intervention is predicated upon a clear definition of patient expectations in the office setting. SCS is highly unlikely to result in complete pain relief. Recent randomized prospective studies by Burchiel and colleagues define procedural success as 50 % reduction in painful leg and back symptoms, finding a positive result in 55 % of patients at 1 year [27]. These findings generally correlate with most modern studies that show that up to 60 % of patients obtain 50 % relief in painful leg and back symptoms [7, 28–33]. A more in-depth discussion of the usage of SCS will be outlined in Chaps. 15 and 16 in this text.

Epidural Injections

Epidural injections for axial LBP in the absence of a localizing finding on MRI can be confirmatory of pathology when followed by symptomatic relief. The route of approach is most commonly interlaminar, and less often transforaminal. However, epidural injections of either anesthetics or in combination with local anesthetics are utilized to provide symptomatic relief of LBP rather than as a diagnostic measure. A positive response from an injection often leads to significant pain reduction and ultimately a delay in the need for surgery, or in some cases obviates the need for additional treatment measures. Injections of glucocorticoids in the epidural space are thought to reduce inflammation of the nerve root, and ultimately pain. Addition of local anesthetics is thought to provide additive benefit by blockage of nociceptive afferent pathways [34, 35]. Evidence in the literature surrounding the use of epidural steroid injections for spinal stenosis is by way of level II and III studies, and no well-designed, randomized, prospective placebo-controlled studies exist [36]. Most recently, a randomized double-blind trial comparing epidural injection of anesthetics with or without glucocorticoids found no additional benefit at 6 weeks with the addition of glucocorticoids [37]. Ultimately, many surgeons require a trial period of analgesic medication, physical therapy, and interventional techniques prior to the consideration of surgery in the absence of any urgent findings on exam or radiographic studies.

Summary

Not all surgical indications are due to encroachment of the neural elements requiring decompression. The increased use of a number of less invasive alternative therapies prior to or in place of surgical decompression such as facet and epidural injections, spinal cord stimulation, radiofrequency neurolysis, and intrathecal pain pump placement serve as evidence of the efficacy of these therapies in treating different modalities of back pain. The key to triage is through an appropriate algorithm to diagnose different pain generators of the spine.

References

1. Andersson GB. Epidemiological features of chronic low-back pain. Lancet. 1999; 354(9178):581–5.
2. Cassidy JD. Saskatchewan health and back pain survey. Spine. 1998;23(17):1923.
3. Cassidy JD, Carroll LJ, Cote P. The Saskatchewan health and back pain survey. The prevalence of low back pain and related disability in Saskatchewan adults. Spine. 1998;23(17):1860–6. discussion 7.
4. Anderson VC, Israel Z. Failed back surgery syndrome. Curr Rev Pain. 2000;4(2):105–11.
5. BenDebba M, Torgerson WS, Boyd RJ, Dawson EG, Hardy RW, Robertson JT, et al. Persistent low back pain and sciatica in the United States: treatment outcomes. J Spinal Disord Tech. 2002;15(1):2–15.
6. Long DM, BenDebba M, Torgerson WS, Boyd RJ, Dawson EG, Hardy RW, et al. Persistent back pain and sciatica in the United States: patient characteristics. J Spinal Disord. 1996;9(1):40–58.
7. Izzo R, Popolizio T, D'Aprile P, Muto M. Spinal pain. Eur J Radiol. 2015.
8. Manchikanti L, Singh V, Falco FJ, Cash KA, Pampati V. Evaluation of lumbar facet joint nerve blocks in managing chronic low back pain: a randomized, double-blind, controlled trial with a 2-year follow-up. Int J Med Sci. 2010;7(3):124–35.
9. Datta S, Lee M, Falco FJ, Bryce DA, Hayek SM. Systematic assessment of diagnostic accuracy and therapeutic utility of lumbar facet joint interventions. Pain Physician. 2009;12(2):437–60.
10. Falco FJ, Manchikanti L, Datta S, Sehgal N, Geffert S, Onyewu O, et al. An update of the systematic assessment of the diagnostic accuracy of lumbar facet joint nerve blocks. Pain Physician. 2012;15(6):E869–907.
11. Manchikanti L, Boswell MV, Singh V, Pampati V, Damron KS, Beyer CD. Prevalence of facet joint pain in chronic spinal pain of cervical, thoracic, and lumbar regions. BMC Musculoskelet Disord. 2004;5:15.

12. Manchikanti L, Manchikanti KN, Pampati V, Brandon DE, Giordano J. The prevalence of facet-joint-related chronic neck pain in postsurgical and nonpostsurgical patients: a comparative evaluation. Pain Pract. 2008;8(1):5–10.
13. Manchikanti L, Pampati V, Baha AG, Fellows B, Damron KS, Barnhill RC. Contribution of facet joints to chronic low back pain in postlumbar laminectomy syndrome: a controlled comparative prevalence evaluation. Pain Physician. 2001;4(2):175–80.
14. Manchikanti L, Pampati V, Fellows B, Bakhit CE. Prevalence of lumbar facet joint pain in chronic low back pain. Pain Physician. 1999;2(3):59–64.
15. Manchikanti L, Pampati V, Rivera J, Fellows B, Beyer C, Damron K. Role of facet joints in chronic low back pain in the elderly: a controlled comparative prevalence study. Pain Pract. 2001;1(4):332–7.
16. Manchikanti L, Pampati V, Bakhit CE, Rivera JJ, Beyer CD, Damron KS, et al. Effectiveness of lumbar facet joint nerve blocks in chronic low back pain: a randomized clinical trial. Pain Physician. 2001;4(1):101–17.
17. Manchikanti L, Singh V, Falco FJ, Cash KA, Pampati V. Lumbar facet joint nerve blocks in managing chronic facet joint pain: one-year follow-up of a randomized, double-blind controlled trial: Clinical Trial NCT00355914. Pain Physician. 2008;11(2):121–32.
18. Nath S, Nath CA, Pettersson K. Percutaneous lumbar zygapophysial (Facet) joint neurotomy using radiofrequency current, in the management of chronic low back pain: a randomized double-blind trial. Spine. 2008;33(12):1291–7. discussion 8.
19. Dreyfuss P, Halbrook B, Pauza K, Joshi A, McLarty J, Bogduk N. Efficacy and validity of radiofrequency neurotomy for chronic lumbar zygapophysial joint pain. Spine. 2000;25(10):1270–7.
20. Carette S, Marcoux S, Truchon R, Grondin C, Gagnon J, Allard Y, et al. A controlled trial of corticosteroid injections into facet joints for chronic low back pain. N Engl J Med. 1991;325(14):1002–7.
21. Schulte TL, Pietila TA, Heidenreich J, Brock M, Stendel R. Injection therapy of lumbar facet syndrome: a prospective study. Acta Neurochir. 2006;148(11):1165–72. discussion 72.
22. Schwarzer AC, Aprill CN, Derby R, Fortin J, Kine G, Bogduk N. The prevalence and clinical features of internal disc disruption in patients with chronic low back pain. Spine. 1995;20(17):1878–83.
23. Bydon M, De la Garza-Ramos R, Macki M, Baker A, Gokaslan AK, Bydon A. Lumbar fusion versus nonoperative management for treatment of discogenic low back pain: a systematic review and meta-analysis of randomized controlled trials. J Spinal Disord Tech. 2014;27(5):297–304.
24. Mannion AF, Brox JI, Fairbank JC. Comparison of spinal fusion and nonoperative treatment in patients with chronic low back pain: long-term follow-up of three randomized controlled trials. Spine J. 2013;13(11):1438–48.
25. De Andres J, Quiroz C, Villanueva V, Valia JC, Lopez Alarcon D, Moliner S, et al. Patient satisfaction with spinal cord stimulation for failed back surgery syndrome. Rev Esp Anestesiol Reanim. 2007;54(1):17–22.
26. Schu S, Slotty PJ, Bara G, von Knop M, Edgar D, Vesper J. A prospective, randomised, double-blind, placebo-controlled study to examine the effectiveness of burst spinal cord stimulation patterns for the treatment of failed back surgery syndrome. Neuromodulation. 2014;17(5):443–50.
27. Burchiel KJ, Anderson VC, Brown FD, Fessler RG, Friedman WA, Pelofsky S, et al. Prospective, multicenter study of spinal cord stimulation for relief of chronic back and extremity pain. Spine. 1996;21(23):2786–94.
28. Broggi G, Servello D, Dones I, Carbone G. Italian multicentric study on pain treatment with epidural spinal cord stimulation. Stereotact Funct Neurosurg. 1994;62(1-4):273–8.
29. Fiume D, Sherkat S, Callovini GM, Parziale G, Gazzeri G. Treatment of the failed back surgery syndrome due to lumbo-sacral epidural fibrosis. Acta Neurochir Suppl. 1995;64:116–8.
30. Hassenbusch SJ, Stanton-Hicks M, Covington EC. Spinal cord stimulation versus spinal infusion for low back and leg pain. Acta Neurochir Suppl. 1995;64:109–15.
31. Meglio M, Cioni B, Visocchi M, Tancredi A, Pentimalli L. Spinal cord stimulation in low back and leg pain. Stereotact Funct Neurosurg. 1994;62(1-4):263–6.

32. North RB, Kidd DH, Lee MS, Piantodosi S. A prospective, randomized study of spinal cord stimulation versus reoperation for failed back surgery syndrome: initial results. Stereotact Funct Neurosurg. 1994;62(1-4):267–72.
33. Ohnmeiss DD, Rashbaum RF, Bogdanffy GM. Prospective outcome evaluation of spinal cord stimulation in patients with intractable leg pain. Spine. 1996;21(11):1344–50. discussion 51.
34. Friedrich JM, Harrast MA. Lumbar epidural steroid injections: indications, contraindications, risks, and benefits. Curr Sports Med Rep. 2010;9(1):43–9.
35. Harrast MA. Epidural steroid injections for lumbar spinal stenosis. Curr Rev Musculoskeletal Med. 2008;1(1):32–8.
36. Bresnahan BW, Rundell SD, Dagadakis MC, Sullivan SD, Jarvik JG, Nguyen H, et al. A systematic review to assess comparative effectiveness studies in epidural steroid injections for lumbar spinal stenosis and to estimate reimbursement amounts. PM R. 2013;5(8):705–14.
37. Friedly JL, Comstock BA, Turner JA, Heagerty PJ, Deyo RA, Sullivan SD, et al. A randomized trial of epidural glucocorticoid injections for spinal stenosis. N Engl J Med. 2014;371(1):11–21.

Chapter 3
Failed Back Surgery Syndrome

Youngwon Youn, Heather C. Smith, and Julie G. Pilitsis

Key Points

- FBSS is not only a major health concern for patients, but also a major socioeconomic burden to society.
- FBSS encompasses a heterogeneous patient population and is multifactorial including biological, social, and economic influences.
- The main etiologies of FBSS can be broken down into preoperative, intraoperative, and postoperative factors.
- FBSS has been reported to occur in up to 40 % of those patients undergoing spinal surgery and is therefore a common and treatable entity within one's spinal practice.
- Preoperative patient mental health status has proven to be a significant predictor of poorer surgical outcomes.
- After a thorough history and physical exam, advanced imaging including MRI with gadolinium, flexion/extension X-rays, and CT can be beneficial.
- The use of interventional pain therapies earlier in the treatment paradigm carries the highest likelihood of success in treating FBSS.

Y. Youn, B.A. • H.C. Smith, B.A. • J.G. Pilitsis, M.D., Ph.D. (✉)
AMC Neurosurgery Group, Albany Medical College,
47 New Scotland Ave., Albany, NY 12208, USA
e-mail: youngwonyoun@gmail.com; smith.heather.2017@gmail.com; jpilitsis@yahoo.com

© Springer International Publishing Switzerland 2016
S.M. Falowski, J.E. Pope (eds.), *Integrating Pain Treatment into Your Spine Practice*, DOI 10.1007/978-3-319-27796-7_3

Introduction, Risk Factors, and Patient Selection

Introduction

Failed back surgery syndrome (FBSS) is persistent or recurring low back pain following one or more spine surgeries and is reported to have an incidence rate of 10 to 40 % [1, 2]. Today, FBSS comprises a notable component of the worldwide epidemic of chronic pain. Specifically, chronic low back pain is estimated to affect 37 % of the general adult population with a 60–80 % lifetime prevalence [3]. These startling numbers demonstrate the extent to which chronic low back pain impacts our society. The etiology of FBSS is driven by a complex relationship of not only biological and psychological factors, but also social and economic.

Etiology and Risk Factors

FBSS is a complex syndrome that is multifactorial. Here we examine the possible preoperative, intraoperative, and postoperative causes (Fig. 3.1).

Patient Selection and Preoperative Factors

Patient selection for the original spine surgery is of the utmost importance in preventing FBSS. It is essential that the proper operation is offered for the correct condition and that patients have reasonable expectations of their surgery. Herniated discs, spinal stenosis, foraminal stenosis, and unstable spondylolisthesis are straight-forward indications. Less commonly, tumors, infection, and/or congenital issues

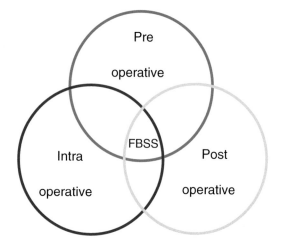

Fig. 3.1 Major contributing factors of failed back surgery syndrome

such as a tethered cord and scoliosis may be present and warrant operation. Other conditions may be approached differently from surgeon to surgeon and often have higher patient dissatisfaction rates and success.

Additional preoperative factors that affect surgical outcome include revision surgery and insufficient candidate screening. In patients who had multiple revisions, the rate of epidural fibrosis and instability increased to greater than 60 % [4]. Additionally, patients must be counseled about reasonable expectations and informed that surgery will not resolve all of their symptoms. Proper counseling of expectations for an initial spine surgery may dramatically reduce the rate of FBSS [5]. For the remaining cases, it is important to ascertain what pain complaint remains following surgery when thinking of further treatment outcomes.

The patient's psychological status is also an important preoperative factor that can strongly impact surgical outcome. It has been shown that depression and anxiety correlate with poorer outcomes [6]. Thus, the patient's ability to cope with stress plays a paramount role in determining who will respond better to surgery. Pain questionnaires used to screen patients include the Pain Catastrophizing Scale (PCS) as well as the Minnesota Multiphasic Personality Inventory (MMPI). The PCS score has been shown to significantly correlate with patients' postoperative pain scores [7]. In addition, the MMPI-2 was shown to be a predictor of implantation status, showing that personality traits or disorders affect the decision-making process for therapy [8]. Unfortunately, economic and social factors also affect psychological status. Patients who are involved in the worker's compensation and/or the litigation process may have less motivation to improve [9]. Another factor that has been found to affect surgical outcome is the weight of the patient. Patients who had normal body mass indices (BMI) were found to have higher scores on emotional well-being scales as well as better perceptions of their disease than those who were obese (BMI>25) [10–12].

Intraoperative Factors

Once an appropriately selected patient reaches the operating room for the correct procedure, other patient and surgical factors may predispose the patient to poorer outcomes. These include modifiable risk factors, such as smoking status, diabetes, and morbid obesity. Smoking is well known to impede fusion and wound healing and some surgeons refuse to perform these surgeries until the patient quits [11, 13, 14]. Additionally, diabetes and obesity significantly increase the risk for surgical site infections (SSI) and perioperative complications [15]. In diabetics, it is essential to ensure that their disease is as well controlled as possible with the help of their endocrinologist and/or primary care physician prior to surgery. Obesity often leads to longer dissection and surgery time which increases the risk for infection and deep vein thrombosis [16]. Other comorbidities related to the spine also need to be accounted for such as immunosuppression, rheumatoid arthritis, renal disease, and osteoporosis/osteopenia. All are associated with higher rates of major complications

[15, 17–19]. Obesity may also necessitate changing routines in the operating room through the use of different tables or retractor systems that are less familiar to the surgeon [20].

Sometimes, findings intraoperatively may result in a less than ideal outcome. Specifically, multiple preoperative epidural steroid injections (ESI) can lead to scarring and difficulty with nerve root retraction [21, 22]. Calcified discs are often harder to remove and may result in greater root retraction and thus postoperative numbness and weakness [23].

Suboptimal surgical technique may also lead to postoperative issues. These include over-distraction of the disc space during fusion, irritation of the nerve roots, and inadequate or overly aggressive decompression [24]. Despite the shift toward more minimally invasive techniques in the past decade, there is no data suggesting lower rates of FBSS [25, 26]. Lastly, it is of course essential to ensure that the surgery was performed at the right level, and that the overall aim of surgery was accomplished by obtaining pre-, intra-, and postoperative imaging [27, 28].

Postoperative Factors

Postoperative impediments to outcome may be due to patient, surgical, or disease factors. Patients may not be compliant with postoperative management. Often bracing or restrictions are implemented and patients do not comply. Though the use of bracing is often controversial, the patient who is noncompliant is likely to be involved in a series of activities that may hinder their surgical outcome. We often instruct patients that they have one chance to heal and should therefore adhere to activity restrictions for the designated length of time. It is their responsibility to take ownership of their health. Patients who are committed to their recovery and doing the right thing such as not smoking, losing weight, and participating in physical therapy when indicated have better outcomes [29–31].

Despite the surgeon and the patient's best work however, complications do occur. Most commonly, an infection or cerebrospinal fluid (CSF) leak can present in the perioperative period. CSF leaks not only predispose the patient to more infections, but also cause headaches, photophobia, nausea, diplopia, and tinnitus [32, 33]. Because SSIs may lead to deeper infections and more serious problems when left unrecognized, these issues must be handled promptly with rapid evaluation of the patient at the onset of signs or symptoms. Additionally, recurrent disc herniations are most common in the initial postoperative period [34]. Patients who have recurrent radiculopathy after a period of relief should be assessed clinically and with imaging.

Disease progression may lead to issues in long-term follow-up. These include the development of scarring (epidural fibrosis, arachnoiditis), anatomical instability, and adjacent level disease. Epidural fibrosis may contribute to persistent pain felt by up to 36 % of FBSS patients due to the tethering of nerve roots [1, 35]. Postsurgical fibrosis at the nerve roots was found to be associated with a higher incidence of recurrent pain following surgery. In a randomized, double-blind clinical trial, patients with extensive peridural scarring were 3.2 times more likely to experience recurrent pain than those with less fibrosis [36]. The researchers suggested that the encasement of the nerve roots with fibrotic tissue was causing pain by increasing neural tension, impairing axoplasmic transport, and constricting blood supply [36]. Perineural scarring often is hyperintense on MRI with gadolinium as opposed to recurrent disc which is hypo- or iso-intense. Additionally, a loss of disc height and anatomic stability after a discectomy can lead to vertical stenosis and compression of nerve roots [28]. This puts patients at risk for foraminal stenosis, disc herniation, or instability [37]. In the long term, adjacent segment disease (ASD) may occur due to hypermobility and increased biomechanic stress on the adjacent segments [38]. It is important to note that FBSS includes all patients with pain after surgery in either the back or the leg or both. Thus, it is likely that some cases of FBSS are really just the natural course of the disease, rather than a failure of surgery as the name implies. It is important to realize that a technically accurate and well-performed surgery does not guarantee success in terms of pain management, as surgical indications for surgery can stem from neurological compromise, as well as prevention of deterioration.

Diagnosis and Treatment

History and Physical Examination

To diagnose FBSS, it is essential to recognize whether the symptoms that prompted the original surgery have been effectively treated. Patients either do or do not improve after the first surgery. Reasons for no improvement include psychological pain, sequestrated missed fragments, infection, wrong initial diagnosis, and suboptimal surgical technique. Some of these factors are amendable to repeat surgery, while some are not. In patients who gain temporary relief and then develop a recurrence of pain, other diagnoses should be entertained. Adjacent level disease, iatrogenic instability, nonunion, and recurrent disc herniation are often amendable to further surgery. Another subset of patients develops fibrosis, complex regional pain syndrome, or neuritis [39]. This group of patients, as well as the patients who received inadequate relief of symptoms despite a good surgical outcome, comprises the majority of FBSS patients.

When evaluating the FBSS patient, the physician should first determine if there was an adequate decrease in pain after surgery or not, thus limiting the differential [39]. The pain itself should be carefully categorized—Is it axial pain isolated to the lower back that worsens with standing? Is it radicular pain shooting down the leg? Are there signs of spinal stenosis-numbness and weakness with walking that improves with bending over? Is the pain presenting the same as before surgery or is this a new type of pain? Is there a new pattern of numbness or weakness? Does the pain localize to the same level as the surgical intervention or is there more diffuse involvement? What is the pain's quality-stabbing and shooting (nociceptive) or burning and aching (neuropathic)? Has the quality of pain changed?

Physical examination in the case of FBSS should also be thorough. Decreased strength and hyperalgesia in specific dermatomes should be noted. It is imperative to differentiate between true chronic pain from decreased flexibility and discomfort from persistent postsurgical pain. In these situations, the patient may regain more function with orthotics and physical rehabilitation than additional medical and invasive management procedures [28].

Advanced Imaging

Advances in radiographic imaging have allowed for the identification of causes of FBSS in 94–95 % of patients [40, 41]. Certain imaging techniques are better suited than others for specific causes.

1. **Plain radiographic imaging:** A basic standing X-ray with flexion and extension of the spine allows for evaluation of alignment, degeneration, and stability of the spine [5]. These are notably valuable for diagnosis of pseudoarthrosis, and instability [39], and confirmation of optimal hardware placement.
2. **Magnetic resonance imaging (MRI):** With few exceptions, MRI is the diagnostic imaging modality of choice—allowing for evaluation of soft tissue, bone marrow, and intraspinal contents [5, 28]. Contrast-enhanced MRI is required in patients who have undergone surgery to differentiate between scarring and persistent disease and to confirm that the aim of surgery was accomplished [5]. MRI imaging should be immediately ordered for patients with risks for spinal infection (new onset of low back pain with fever and history of IV drug abuse), signs of cauda equina syndrome (urine retention, fecal incontinence, saddle anesthesia), or severe neurological deficits [42].
3. **Computer-assisted tomography (CT):** CT with multiplanar reconstruction is preferred for patients with pedicle screws or fusions [41, 43, 44] to rule out pseudoarthrosis and check hardware while limiting effects of artifact. CT myelography is indicated for patients with ferromagnetic metal alloy instrumentation to allow for adequate image quality and resolution, or if MRI is contraindicated for the individual patient.
4. **Diagnostic injections:** Diagnosis of facet joint arthropathy, sacroiliac joint (SIJ) pain, and foraminal or central stenosis can be confirmed and localized with diagnostic injections, such as intra-articular injections, nerve root blocks, and transforaminal/interlaminar epidural steroid injections.

Treatment of FBSS

The general goals of treatment include the following: (1) treat the cause when possible; (2) decrease pain and inflammation; (3) maximize neuromuscular and musculoskeletal function; and (4) stop the progression of disability [28, 39]. Similar to treatment of other chronic pain syndromes, treatment of FBSS entails a multidisciplinary approach, incorporating physical therapy, psychological counseling, medication, and interventional procedures when necessary [5]; holistic treatments such as chiropractic care, acupuncture, and biofeedback therapy also provide benefit [45].

Traditional pharmacologic management includes:

1. Nonsteroidal anti-inflammatory drugs or acetaminophen.
2. Muscle relaxants, such as cyclobenzaprine.
3. Antispastic medications, such as baclofen or tizanidine.
4. Antidepressants, such as tricyclic antidepressants, serotonin-norepinephrine reuptake inhibitors, or selective serotonin reuptake inhibitors.
5. Antiepileptics (gabapentin).
6. Tramadol.
7. Opioids—although opioid-induced hyperalgesia is likely under-recognized and under-reported [28]. It is the authors' recommendation that the use of long-term opioid use for this patient population is not a viable option.

Concurrent with pharmacologic management other interventional pain procedures may be employed, such as epidural injections, branch blocks, radiofrequency ablation, and spinal cord stimulation (SCS) [5, 28]. Specific treatment for chronic pain and indications will be discussed in further detail in later chapters; however, it is important to note that earlier interventions have been noted to have higher success rates for the treatment of chronic pain. A recent meta-regression and stratified meta-analysis performed by Taylor and colleagues [46] found a longer duration of pain to correlate with less pain relief provided by SCS—suggesting superiority of earlier intervention [46]. This applies to less invasive therapies as well, such as physical therapy [47]. Early intervention can also reduce the amount of sick time the patient uses in the future [48]. Consequently, this evidence suggests the importance of early intervention.

Summary

With spinal surgeries continuing to rise, the incidence of FBSS has been reported to be as high as 40 %, posing a significant economic burden on society. As a complex multifactorial pain syndrome, FBSS has many components including pre-, intra-, and postoperative factors, as well as psychological and socioeconomic elements.

A careful history and physical exam is essential in diagnosing FBSS. Imaging options also serve as important diagnostic tools and include plain radiographs, MRI, and CT. Once diagnosis has been established, the goals of treatment are to treat the underlying cause when possible, decrease pain and inflammation, and maximize function as well as slow the progression of disability. This has largely been accomplished by a range of pharmacological medication, injections, and SCS with earlier intervention and recognition leading to higher success rates with treatment.

References

1. Chan C, Peng P. Failed back surgery syndrome. Pain Med. 2011;12:577–606.
2. North RB, Campbell JN, James CS, et al. Failed back surgery syndrome: 5-year follow-up in 102 patients undergoing repeated operation. Neurosurgery. 1991;28:685–90.
3. Schmidt CO, Raspe H, Pfingsten M. Back pain in the German adult population: prevalence, severity, and socio-demographic correlates in a multiregional survey. Spine. 2007;32:2005–11.
4. Fritsch EW, Heisel J, Rupp S. The failed back surgery syndrome—reasons, intraoperative findings, and long term results: a report of 182 operative treatments. Spine. 1996;21:626–33.
5. Hussain A, Erdek M. Interventional pain management for failed back surgery syndrome. Pain Pract. 2014;14(1):64–78.
6. Trief PM, Grant W, Fredrickson B. A prospective study of psychological predictors of lumbar surgery outcome. Spine (Phila Pa 1976). 2000;25(20):2616–21.
7. Granot M, Ferber S. The roles of pain catastrophizing and anxiety in the prediction of postoperative pain intensity: a prospective study. Clin J Pain. 2005;21(5):439–45.
8. Ruchinskas R, O'Grady T. Psychological variables predict decisions regarding implantation of a spinal cord stimulator. Neuromodulation. 2000;3(4):183–9.
9. KleKamp J, McCarty E, Sprengler DM. Results for elective lumbar discectomy for patients involved in the worker's compensation system. J Spinal Disord. 1998;11:277–82.
10. Jitta DJ, DeJongste MJ, Kliphuis CM, Staal MJ. Multimorbidity, the predominant predictor of quality-of-life, following successful spinal cord stimulation for angina pectoris. Neuromodulation. 2011;14(1):13–8.
11. Sloan A, Hussain I, Maqsood M, Eremin O, El-Sheemy M. The effects of smoking on fracture healing. Surgeon. 2010;8(2):111–6.
12. Sørensen LT. Wound healing and infection in surgery: the pathophysiological impact of smoking, smoking cessation, and nicotine replacement therapy: a systematic review. Ann Surg. 2012;355(6):1069–79.
13. Lau D, Chou D, Ziewacz JE, Mummaneni PV. The effects of smoking on perioperative outcomes and pseudarthrosis following anterior cervical corpectomy: clinical article. J Neurosurg Spine. 2014;21(4):547–58.
14. Tamaki J, Iki M, Fujita Y, Kouda K, Yura A, Kadowaki E, Sato Y, Moon JS, Tomioka K, Okamoto N, Kurumatani N. Impact of smoking on bone mineral density and bone metabolism in elderly men: the Fujiwara-kyo Osteoporosis Risk in Men (FORMEN) study. Osteoporos Int. 2011;22(1):133–41.
15. Pull ter Gunne AF, Cohen DB. Incidence, prevalence, and analysis of risk factors for surgical site infection following adult spinal surgery. Spine (Phila Pa 1976). 2009;34(13):1422–8.
16. Childs BR, Nahm NJ, Dolenc AJ, Vallier HA. Obesity is associated with more complications and longer hospital stays after orthopaedic trauma. J Orthop Trauma. 2015;29:504–9.
17. Lehman Jr RA, Kang DG, Wagner SC. Management of osteoporosis in spine surgery. J Am Acad Orthop Surg. 2015;23(4):253–63.
18. Martin CT, Pugely AJ, Gao Y, Mendoza-Lattes SA, Weinstein SL. The impact of renal impairment on short term morbidity risk following lumbar spine surgeries. Spine (Phila Pa 1976). 2015;40:909–16.
19. Mesfin A, El Dafrawy MH, Jain A, Hassanzadeh H, Kostuik JP, Lemma MA, Kebaish KM. Surgical outcomes of long spinal fusions for scoliosis in adult patients with rheumatoid arthritis. J Neurosurg Spine. 2015;22(4):367–73. doi:10.3171/2014.10.SPINE14365.
20. DeMaria EJ, Carmody BJ. Perioperative management of special populations: obesity. Surg Clin North Am. 2005;85(6):1283–9.
21. Murthy N, Geske J, Shelerud R, Wald J, Diehn F, Thielen K, Kaufmann T, Morris J, Lehman V, Amrami K, Carter R, Maus T. The effectiveness of repeat lumbar transforaminal epidural steroid injections. Pain Med. 2014;15(10):1686–94.
22. Radcliff K, Kepler C, Hilibrand A, Rihn J, Zhao W, Lurie J, Tosteson T, Vaccaro A, Albert T, Weinstein J. Epidural steroid injections are associated with less improvement in patients with

lumbar spinal stenosis: a subgroup analysis of the Spine Patient Outcomes Research Trial. Spine (Phila Pa 1976). 2013;38(4):279–91.

23. Yang HS, Chen DY, Yuan W, Yang LL, Tsai N, Lin QS. Paresis associated with aconuresis caused by intervertebral disc calcification at c7-t1: a case report and review of the literature. Spine (Phila Pa 1976). 2010;35(10):E434–9.

24. Phillips FM, Cunningham B. Managing chronic pain of spinal origin after lumbar surgery. The role of decompressive surgery. Spine. 2002;27:2547–53.

25. Gempt J, Jonek M, Ringel F, Preuß A, Wolf P, Ryang Y. Long-term follow-up of standard microdiscectomy versus minimal access surgery for lumbar disc herniations. Acta Neurochir. 2013;155(12):2333–8.

26. Ryang YM, Oertel MF, Mayfrank L, Gilsbach JM, Rohde V. Standard open microdiscectomy versus minimal access trocar microdiscectomy: results of a prospective randomized study. Neurosurgery. 2008;62(1):174–82.

27. Epstein NE. Foraminal and far lateral lumbar disc herniations: surgical alternatives. Spinal Cord. 2002;40:491–500.

28. Shapiro CM. The failed back surgery syndrome: pitfalls surrounding evaluation and treatment. Phys Med Rehabil Clin N Am. 2014;25(2):319–40.

29. Behrend C, Prasarn M, Coyne E, Horodyski M, Wright J, Rechtine GR. Smoking cessation related to improved patient-reported pain scores following spinal care. J Bone Joint Surg Am. 2012;94(23):2161–6.

30. De Groef A, Van Kampen M, Dieltjens E, Christiaens MR, Neven P, Geraerts I, Devoogdt N. Effectiveness of postoperative physical therapy for upper-limb impairments after breast cancer treatment: a systematic review. Arch Phys Med Rehabil. 2015;15:00010–6.

31. Skolasky RL, Mackenzie EJ, Wegener ST, Riley III LH. Patient activation and functional recovery in persons undergoing spine surgery. J Bone Joint Surg Am. 2011;93(18):1665–71.

32. Bendersky D, Yampolsky C. Is spinal cord stimulation safe? A review of its complications. World Neurosurg. 2014;82(6):1359–68.

33. Eldrige JS, Weingarten TN, Rho RH. Management of cerebral spinal fluid leak complicating spinal cord stimulator implantation. Pain Pract. 2006;6(4):285–8.

34. Matsumoto M, Watanabe K, Hosogane N, Tsuji T, Ishii K, Nakamura M, Chiba K, Toyama Y. Recurrence of lumbar disc herniation after microendoscopic discectomy. J Neurol Surg A Cent Eur Neurosurg. 2013;74(4):222–7.

35. Coskun E, Suzer T, Topuz O. Relationships between epidural fibrosis, pain, disability, and psychological factors after lumbar disc surgery. Eur J Spine. 2000;9:218–23.

36. Ross JS, Robertson JT, Frederickson RC, Petrie JL, Obuchowski N, Modic MT, deTribolet N. Association between peridural scar and recurrent radicular pain after lumbar discectomy: magnetic resonance evaluation. ADCON-L European Study Group. Neurosurgery. 1996;38(4):e.g. 45.

37. Kumar MN, Baklanov A, Chopin D. Correlation between sagittal plan changes and adjacent level degeneration following lumbar spine fusion. Eur Spin J. 2001;10:314–9.

38. Hikata T, Kamata M, Furukawa M. Risk factors for adjacent segment disease after posterior lumbar interbody fusion and efficacy of simultaneous decompression surgery for symptomatic adjacent segment disease. J Spinal Disord Tech. 2014;27(2):70–5.

39. Walker BF. Failed back surgery syndrome. COSMIG Rev. 1992;1(1):3–6.

40. Slipman CW, Shin CH, Patel RK, et al. Etiologies of failed back surgery syndrome. Pain Med. 2002;3(3):200–14. discussion 214–7.

41. Waguespack A, Schofferman J, Slosar P, Reynolds J. Etiology of long-term failures of lumbar spine surgery. Pain Med. 2002;3(1):18–22.

42. Chou R, Qaseem A, Owens DK, et al. Diagnostic imaging for low back pain: advice for high-value health care from the American College of Physicians. Ann Intern Med. 2011;154:181.

43. Guyer RD, Patterson M, Ohnmeiss DD. Failed back surgery syndrome: diagnostic evaluation. J Am Acad Orthop Surg. 2006;14(9):534–43.

44. Herzog RJ, Marcotte PJ. Assessment of spinal fusion. Critical evaluation of imaging techniques. Spine (Phila Pa 1976). 1996;21(9):1114–8.

45. Furlan AD, Yazdi F, Tsertsvadze A, Gross A, Van Tulder M, Santaguida L, Cherkin D, Gagnier J, Ammendolia C, Ansari MT, Ostermann T, Dryden T, Doucette S, Skidmore B, Daniel R, Tsouros S, Weeks L, Galipeau J. Complementary and alternative therapies for back pain II. Evid Rep Technol Assess (Full Rep). 2010;194:1–764.
46. Taylor RS, Desai MJ, Rigoard P, Taylor RJ. Predictors of pain relief following spinal cord stimulation in chronic back and leg pain and failed back surgery syndrome: a systematic review and meta-regression analysis. Pain Pract. 2014;14(6):489–505.
47. Wand BM, Bird C, Mcauley JH, Doré CJ, Macdowell M, De souza LH. Early intervention for the management of acute low back pain: a single-blind randomized controlled trial of biopsychosocial education, manual therapy, and exercise. Spine. 2004;29(21):2350–6.
48. Hagen EM, Eriksen HR, Ursin H. Does early intervention with a light mobilization program reduce long-term sick leave for low back pain? Spine. 2000;25(15):1973–6.

Chapter 4
Cervical Pain Syndromes

Bryan C. Hoelzer

Key Points

- Cervical pain syndromes are common.
- There are numerous potential pain generators in the cervical spine.
- There is not an isolated physical exam test or imaging modality that will allow for the correct diagnosis of the etiology of cervical pain.
- By carefully applying the history, physical exam, imagining, and diagnostic studies the source of pain can typically be identified.
- There are many minimally invasive procedures that offer patients hope of improving from cervical pain.

Introduction

Pain originating in the cervical spine is a common patient complaint. In the general population, the life time prevalence of neck pain is estimated at 30 to 50 % [1–3]. Furthermore, 1.5 to 1.8 % of adults seek treatment for neck pain annually [4]. While neck pain is quite common in the general population identifying the pain generator can be elusive and without a clear etiology formulating the best treatment course may be difficult [5]. For the purposes of this chapter cervical pain is defined as pain originating in the cervical spine with or without radicular features.

When seeing a patient with cervical pain the clinician's first priority is to review any symptoms consistent with more serious underlying diseases. The so-called red

B.C. Hoelzer, M.D. (✉)
Anesthesiology and Pain Medicine, Mayo Clinic,
200 First St., SW, Rochester, MN 55905, USA
e-mail: hoelzer.bryan@mayo.edu

© Springer International Publishing Switzerland 2016
S.M. Falowski, J.E. Pope (eds.), *Integrating Pain Treatment into Your Spine Practice*, DOI 10.1007/978-3-319-27796-7_4

flag symptoms (Table 4.1) give clues to the clinician when a more systemic evaluation is warranted [5, 6]. Cervical myelopathy refers to direct compression to the cervical spine most typically from a combination of degenerative changes to the uncovertebral joints, facet joints, hypertrophy of the ligamentum flavum, and herniation of the cervical disks. Symptoms include pain in the neck, shoulders, or arms, gait instability, numbness and weakness in the upper and/or lower extremities, and changes in bowel or bladder function [5]. Progression of these symptoms warrants immediate surgical evaluation. Once a more serious underlying disease has been ruled out attention can be focused on more benign, but still very distressing to the patient, causes of neck pain.

The cervical spine is a complex anatomical structure with important interactions between muscle, disk, bone, nerve, blood vessel, ligaments, and joints (Fig. 4.1). As a result there are a number of potential pain generators in the neck. While much is known about the anatomy of the neck very little is known about the mechanisms of

Table 4.1 Red flags for possible serious underlying disease

Fever or chills	Trauma
Unexplained weight loss	Osteoporosis
History of cancer	History of ankylosing spondylitis
History of intravenous drug abuse	Bowel of bladder changes
Recent infection	Upper of lower extremity spasticity
Immunosuppression	Upper of lower extremity weakness
History of inflammatory arthritis	

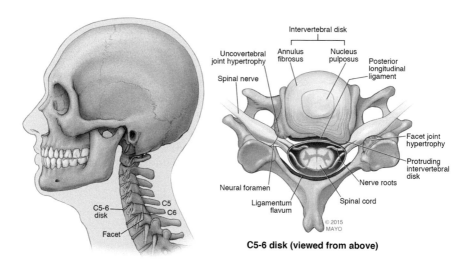

Fig. 4.1 Medical illustration of a sagittal and axial view of the cervical spine at the C5-6 level. Note the potential for neuroforaminal stenosis from uncovertebral joint hypertrophy, disk herniation, or facet joint hypertrophy. Reprinted with permission from "Mayo 2015"

Table 4.2 Common and uncommon causes of cervical pain

Common	Uncommon
Facet osteoarthritis	Vertebral tumors
Discogenic neck pain	Discitis
Myofascial pain	Septic arthritis
Disk herniation	Osteomyelitis
Neuroforaminal stenosis	Inflammatory arthropathies
Shoulder disease	Fractures
	Vascular disease

cervical pain [4, 6]. Despite this complexity, known etiologies of neck pain have been identified and studied [3, 7–15]. It should be pointed out that degenerative changes or anomalies seen on diagnostic imaging do not always equate to pain. It is the clinician's job to overlay the history, physical exam, imaging studies, and possibly invasive diagnostic studies to correctly determine the etiology of cervical pain. Once the likely source of pain is identified appropriate treatments can be offered to the patient. This chapter does not cover all sources of cervical pain but focuses on the more common causes including cervical radiculopathy, facet osteoarthritis, discogenic neck pain, myofascial pain, and spondyloarthropathies (Table 4.2). It does not cover trauma, myelopathy, infections, malignancy, or vascular sources of pain as these conditions require more emergent evaluation and are beyond the scope of this chapter.

Cervical Radiculopathy

Incidence and Mechanism

Cervical radicular pain is described as pain originating in the neck with radiation over the posterior shoulder, upper scapular region, arm, and hand. It is characterized by a combination of sensory, motor, and/or reflex impairment of the neck and upper extremities [16]. In order for pain to be present the dorsal root ganglion must also be compressed or irritated [6]. While it is less common than axial neck pain, it is still quite prevalent occurring in 85 out of 100,000 patients annually [17]. It is most common in the sixth decade of life but can affect all adult patients [16]. Non-compressive causes such as diabetic plexopathies, herpes zoster, primary shoulder disease, upper extremity nerve entrapment, and root avulsion account for a small minority of the total cervical radiculopathy but should be included in the differential diagnosis prior to entertaining the more common causes [5, 7]. Over 90 % of cervical radiculopathies result from direct compression or irritation of the cervical nerve root and dorsal root ganglion. Unlike the lumbar spine, the most common causes of cervical nerve root compression are cervical spondylosis followed by cervical disk herniation [7, 18, 19]. In this setting spondylosis refers to the age related changes of the uncovertebral joint, cervical facet joints, intervertebral disks, and ligamentum flavum all of which contribute to neuroforaminal narrowing. Degeneration and hypertrophy in these cervical structures leads to narrowing of the neuro foramen and results in compressive symptoms to the cervical spinal nerve [5].

History and Physical Exam

Patients suffering from a cervical radiculopathy generally describe a sharp, burning, shooting, and/or electric pain located in the neck, shoulder, arm or hand depending on the affected nerve root (Table 4.3) [7]. Of patients presenting with cervical radiculopathy 99 % complained of arm pain, 85 % had sensory deficits, and 80 % complained of neck pain [20]. The lower cervical spinal levels are most common. The C7 nerve root is involved in 45 to 60 % of patients with C6 accounting for 20 to 25 %. The C5 and C8 spinal nerve roots each account for approximately 10 % of the cases [16]. It should be noted that a C6-7 disk herniation will result in a C7 radiculopathy.

Findings on physical exam may include decreased sensation, upper extremity weakness, and hyporeflexia. Provocative maneuvers including the upper limb tension test (ULTT), neck distraction, Spurling test, and the shoulder abduction test increase the clinician's suspicions of a radicular source by exacerbating or relieving the patient's radicular pain. Of the provocative maneuvers the ULTT is the most sensitive for cervical radiculopathy [5, 21–23].

Table 4.3 Neurologic manifestations of cervical radiculopathies

Nerve root	Sensory changes	Muscle weakness	Reflex loss	Pain pattern
C5	Lateral shoulder **Lateral upper arm**	**Deltoid** Biceps Supraspinatus Infraspinatus	Supinator **Biceps**	Neck, medial upper scapular border, shoulder, and lateral upper arm
C6	**Lateral forearm** Thumb Index finger	Biceps Brachioradialis **Wrist extensors**	Biceps **Brachioradialis**	Neck, scapula, shoulder, lateral forearm, and thumb
C7	Posterior forearm **3rd finger**	**Triceps** Wrist flexors Latissimus dorsi Finger extensors	**Triceps**	Neck, medial scapula, posterior forearm, and 3rd finger
C8	Medial forearm **5th finger**	Triceps Thumb flexors **Hand abductors**	None	Neck, medial forearm, and 5th finger

Imaging and Advanced Diagnostics

Plain film radiographs and more advanced imaging modalities for nontraumatic neck pain are rarely helpful and should be reserved for patients with red flag symptoms (Table 4.1) or in patients with pain that last longer than 6 weeks and is unresponsive to conservative treatment [5, 16]. Plain film radiographs offer information regarding congenital abnormalities, disk degeneration, instability, fractures, and sagittal alignment. However, none of these findings, including abnormal curvature, are predictive of more severe underlying diseases [7, 24].

Magnetic resonance images (MRI) is clearly superior to any other imaging modality when assessing changes in the intervertebral disk, nerve root, dorsal root ganglion, spinal cord, the neuro foramen and surrounding soft tissues all of which could account for radicular symptoms (Fig. 4.2), however, there is no direct link between abnormalities seen in these structures and pain. In fact studies have shown abnormal MRI results in 10 to 60 % of asymptomatic patients depending on age [16, 17, 25, 26]. As a result the correct diagnosis of cervical radiculopathy, including the level involved, requires careful layering of all components of the history, physical exam, and imaging studies.

Electromyography (EMG) and nerve conduction tests may be useful when the history, physical exam, and other imaging studies cannot differentiate between a radicular source of pain and other neurological pain generators of the upper extremity (i.e., distal nerve entrapments or plexopathies). In addition, an EMG may be of value when multiple levels of neuroforaminal stenosis are seen on MRI because specific spinal nerve roots can be tested as long as the upper extremity symptoms have been present for greater than 3 weeks [7, 16, 27]. However, mild radiculopathies may have a normal EMG [28].

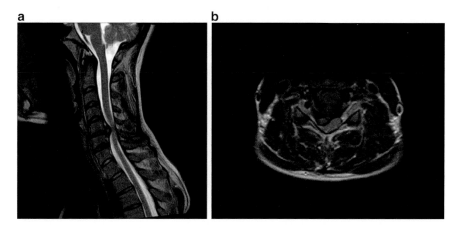

Fig. 4.2 A 42-year-old female with new radicular pain in a right C6 distribution. (**a**) T2 weight sagittal MRI showing a large C-6 disk herniation. (**b**) T2 weighted axial MRI of the same patient showing the disk herniation impinging the right C6 nerve root

Cervical Facets

Incidence and Mechanism

The cervical facet joint is a common source for axial neck pain accounting for 25 to 65 % of patients suffering from neck pain depending on the selection method [29–33]. In patients suffering from chronic neck pain after a known whiplash injury the prevalence of pain coming from one or more cervical facet joint is 54 to 60 % [34, 35]. As a diarthrotic joint it is susceptible to traumatic, occupational, and age related degenerations resulting in its high prevalence [36]. While all levels of the cervical facets can be sources of pain the most common levels are C2-3 and C5-6. In nearly half the patients suffering from cervical fact mediated pain more than one facet joint was involved [37]. Studies have shown that occupation plays a significant rate in developing neck pain and may be secondary to added stress on the facet joints during prolonged flexion or extension [38, 39].

History and Physical Exam

As with cervical radiculopathy a clinician's first responsibility is to rule out any serious underlying disease before establishing the diagnosis of cervical facet pain. Part of this evaluation should include questioning the patient about previous trauma, weight loss, night pain, and history of malignancy. Cervical facet pain has been described as a dull or sharp pain in the posterior lateral and dorsal side of the spinal column with radiation into the scapular region, upper shoulders or head depending on the level affected [6, 36]. In some cases the pain may radiate into the upper arm but should not go distal to the elbow unless the facet hypertrophy is also affecting the neuro foramen. Fortunately, pain from the cervical facet joints often follows a specific and clinically recognizable pattern (Fig. 4.3) [6, 37]. The pain is often exacerbated with rotation, flexion, and neck extension. In fact, patient's first complaint may be pain and stiffness when rotating their neck to look behind them while reversing a car.

The physical exam should include eliminating cervical radiculopathy as well as shoulder pathology as potential pain generators. In addition, a neurologic exam of the upper extremities should be normal in patients with cervical facet disease. Provocative manners that produce pressure and tension on the cervical facets are often helpful. For upper facets (C2-3 and C3-4) rotation of the cervical spine in a flexed position (looking at the floor) may reproduce pain. Movement in the lower facets (C5-6 and C6-7) can be assessed by rotating the cervical spine in an extended position (looking at the ceiling) [36]. In addition, research has demonstrated that pain along the facet column with 4 kg of locally applied pressure is indicative of cervical facet disease [40].

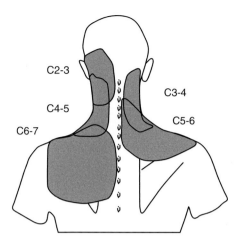

Fig. 4.3 The patterns of referred pain from cervical facet joints. From Cooper G, Bailey B, Bogduk N. Cervical zygapophysial joint pain maps. Pain Med. 2007;8(4):344–53. Reprinted with permission from John Wiley and Sons

Imaging and Advanced Diagnostics

In patients suffering with axial neck pain imaging studies are rarely helpful. Plain film radiographs may exclude tumor, fracture, or other serious systemic disease. In addition, plain films may help establish the degree of degeneration in the cervical facets (Fig. 4.4). While correlation between degeneration seen on imaging and pain symptoms is controversial there are studies showing a relationship between advanced degenerative changes on plain film radiographs and facet mediated pain [36, 41].

Advances in magnetic resonance imaging (MRI) have enabled clinicians to see signs of inflammatory changes in the cervical facet (Fig. 4.4). However, like degeneration in plain film radiographs inflammation does not necessarily correlate to that cervical facet joint(s) being the source of pain. EMG studies are not indicated for axial neck pain.

The most reliable way to establish if the cervical facets are the etiology of a patient's axial neck pain is by performing diagnostic blocks of the medial branches that supply sensory innervation to each joint. It has been verified that the cervical facet joint is innervated via the medial branches of the rami dorsales from the spinal nerves above and below the joint. For example, to confirm the C6-7 facet joint as painful a small amount (0.25 to 0.5 mls) of local anesthetic is injected under image guidance onto the medial branches of the rami dorsales of C5 and C6. Although invasive this modality can be vital in establishing a clear diagnosis and allow the clinician and patient to consider other minimally invasive treat options for cervical facet pain [13, 33, 36, 40, 42].

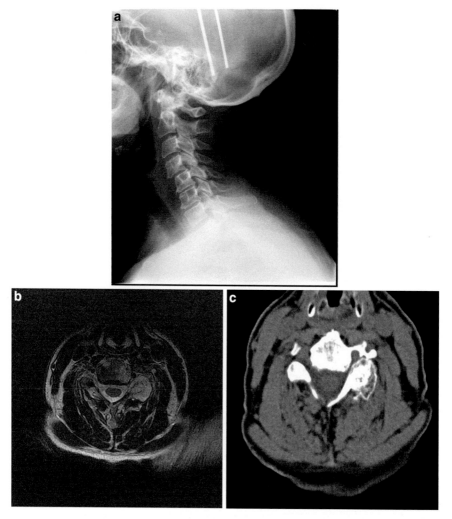

Fig. 4.4 63 year old female with chronic pain located in her mid-left neck without radiation. (**a**) Plain film radiograph showing degenerative changes in the C4-5 joints. (**b**) T2 weighted axial MRI using fast spin echo (FSE) sequencing showing degenerative changes in the left C4-5 facet joint. (**c**) CT scan showing advanced degeneration at the C4-5 level on the left

Cervical Disks

Incidence and Mechanism

The cervical disks are innervated by the sinuvertebral nerves, vertebral nerve, and the cervical sympathetic trunk [43–45]. Degeneration of the cervical disk can result in pain in other areas of the cervical spine (i.e., radiculopathy, uncovertebral joint, and facet joint). However, the cervical disks themselves have been identified as a source of neck pain [46]. The exact incidence of discogenic neck pain is unknown however one study estimated it to be present in 16 % of patients with complaints of neck pain [33].

History and Physical Exam

Patients with neck pain from a discogenic source will complain of a dull aching pain over the midline neck with the level depending on the disk involved. The pain will not radiate unless the disk degeneration has become significant enough to cause nerve root irritation [45]. No physical exam maneuver has been validated to be specific or sensitive for disk mediated pain however, neck distraction may give the examiner some clue that the disk may be involved. Therefore, the history and physical exam center on eliminating other more common sources of neck pain.

Imaging and Advanced Diagnostics

Degeneration of the cervical disks can be seen on plain film radiographs, magnetic resonance images (MRI) and CT scans. As with other sources of neck pain degeneration does not equate to pain. There is some belief that annular tears identified as high intensity zones on T2 weighted MRI images may correlate with discogenic pain. However, fissures have been shown to be a normal part of age related disk changes [45, 47]. In order to correlate degenerative changes seen on imaging with discogenic neck pain cervical discography must be performed [46]. Because the symptoms of cervical disk and facet pain are similar it is recommended that the facet joint (via medial branch blocks) is first evaluated as a source of neck pain prior to commencing cervical discography [33]. When this order is not followed it has been shown that discography will be falsely positive in over 30 % of cases [48].

Electromyography (EMG) and nerve conduction tests are not indicated in cases of isolated cervical disk pain.

Cervical Myalgias

Incidence and Mechanism

It is estimated that up to 55 % of patients evaluated for head and neck pain have a component of myofascial pain [49]. While the exact mechanism of cervical myofascial pain has not been fully discovered it often involves the development of palpable taut muscle fibers known as trigger points [50]. Any muscle of the cervical spine can contribute to neck pain, but the trapezius, levator scapulae, and semispinalis muscles are often involved. Tendonitis of the longus colli muscle is a rare condition that can lead to cervical pain [6]. Polymyalgia rheumatic and fibromyalgia are both systemic diseases that typically have cervical manifestations [6]. In addition, other cervical diseases such as radiculopathy or facet degeneration often coexist with myofascial pain.

History and Physical Exam

Determining a myofascial source of cervical pain involves combining a comprehensive neurological and musculoskeletal exam to exclude deeper causes of pain while identifying specific muscles that have point tenderness and taut muscle fibers to palpation [51]. Cervical myofascial pain often presents as a deep aching sensation and patients use descriptors such as tight, stiff, and dull. Patients will also complain of and demonstrate a decreased range of motion [52]. Questioning may reveal a history of minor trauma, sleep disturbances, psychological stressors, and/or repetitive over use [53]. Muscles spasms may be misinterpreted as radicular symptoms.

Imaging and Advanced Diagnostics

There are no specific imaging or advanced diagnostics studies that are recommended for cervical myalgias, however; magnetic resonance imaging can demonstrate inflammation and edema in the upper longus colli muscle [54].

Cervical Spondyloarthopathies

Incidence and Mechanism

The two most common inflammatory arthritides to affect the spine are rheumatoid arthritis and ankyloses spondylosis. Rheumatoid arthritis preferentially causing changes in the cervical spine while ankylosing spondylitis can involve the cervical, thoracic, and lumbar spine. Although not as common, other inflammatory disorders such as psoriatic arthritis and crystal depositing arthropathies can also involve the cervical spine. In most cases the peripheral manifestations of these disorders are more severe than axial complaints which may result in overlooking their impact on the cervical spine [55]. However, 40 to 85 % of patients with rheumatoid arthritis complain of neck pain secondary to cervical involvement of their rheumatoid arthritis [56, 57].

History and Physical Exam

The most common manifestations of inflammatory arthritis in the cervical spine are basilar invagination, subaxial instability, and atlantoaxial instability [55, 58]. These conditions can present as a combination of radiculopathy, axial pain, and/or cervical myelopathy [55]. There are no specific symptoms a patient suffering with an inflammatory arthritis with cervical involvement will complain of. In patients with a history of inflammatory arthritis a thorough upper and lower neurological exam should be performed to assess for the subtleties of an impending myelopathy. Once serious neurologic involvement is excluded attention can be turned to the causes of cervical pain that have already been described in this chapter.

Imaging and Advanced Diagnostics

Indications for imaging patients with inflammatory arthritis include neurologic dysfunction attributable to cervical cord or nerve root compression, sudden onset of gait instability, new occipital headache, pending surgical procedure involving airway manipulation, and axial neck pain lasting more than 6 weeks [55]. Plain film radiographs including flexion–extension views and odontoid views offer an inexpensive screen for dynamic instability. MRI imaging allows for the detailed evaluation of the ligaments and joint capsules affected by inflammatory arthritis and their effects on the spinal canal [59]. In patients suffering from rheumatoid arthritis a CT scan is superior for evaluating basilar invagination. CT scans also provide information about the bony architecture of the cervical spine [60].

Treatments

While other chapters focus more extensively on the treatment options for cervical pain syndromes this chapter would not be complete without a brief mention of those options. For patients suffering from acute and subacute cervical radiculopathies, epidural steroid injections have been shown to offer temporary relief allowing patients to participate more fully in physical therapy [61]. When the primary pain generator has been identified as the facet joint radiofrequency ablation has been shown to provide significant long-lasting pain relief [42, 62]. For myofascial pain trigger point injections may be beneficial although the evidence for their use is sparse.

For patients suffering from cervical pain that has not responded to the above treatments utilization of spinal cord stimulation may provide significant pain relief. In particular, patients suffering from chronic radiculopathy may benefit most from this therapy [63]. As the technology surrounding spinal cord stimulation evolves and with the emergence of new stimulation options a great portion of patients with cervical pain syndromes from all etiologies may find relief with spinal cord stimulation.

Finally, for patients with severe refractory pain utilization of intrathecal drug delivery systems remains a viable option. These systems are particularly useful in patients with intolerable side effects to systemic opioids, however; their use requires the physician to have extensive experience with both the implantation and maintenance of the system [64].

Summary

Cervical pain syndromes are common among a diverse patient population. Identifying the pain generator can be difficult, however; if a clinician approaches this problem with careful attention to the history, physical exam, and imaging, a diagnosis can be made. Before starting down the path of conservative management, questions aimed at ruling out serious underlying disease must be answered.

References

1. Haldeman SDCMDP, Carroll LJP, Cassidy JDDCPD. The empowerment of people with neck pain: introduction: the bone and joint decade 2000–2010 task force on neck pain and its associated disorders. Spine (Phila Pa 1976). 2008;33 Suppl 4:S8–13.
2. Hogg-Johnson SP, van der Velde GDC, Carroll LJP, Holm LWD, Cassidy JDDCP, Guzman JMDMF, et al. The burden and determinants of neck pain in the general population: results of the bone and joint decade 2000–2010 task force on neck pain and its associated disorders. Spine (Phila Pa 1976). 2008;33 Suppl 4:S39–51.
3. Carroll LJ, Hogg-Johnson S, van der Velde G, Haldeman S, Holm LW, Carragee EJ, et al. Course and prognostic factors for neck pain in the general population: results of the bone and joint decade 2000–2010 task force on neck pain and its associated disorders. Spine (Phila Pa 1976). 2008;33 Suppl 4:S75–82 [Research Support, Non-U.S. Gov't Review].
4. Guzman JMDMF, Haldeman SDCMDP, Carroll LJP, Carragee EJMDF, Hurwitz ELDCP, Peloso PMDMF, et al. Clinical practice implications of the bone and joint decade 2000–2010 task force on neck pain and its associated disorders: from concepts and findings to recommendations. Spine (Phila Pa 1976). 2008;33 Suppl 4:S199–213.
5. Evans G. Identifying and treating the causes of neck pain. Med Clin North Am. 2014;98(3):645–61 [Review].
6. Bogduk N. The anatomy and pathophysiology of neck pain. Phys Med Rehabil Clin N Am. 2011;22(3):367–82, vii [Review].
7. Abbed KM, Coumans JV. Cervical radiculopathy: pathophysiology, presentation, and clinical evaluation. Neurosurgery. 2007;60(1 Suppl 1):S28–34 [Review].
8. Ahn NU, Ahn UM, Ipsen B, An HS. Mechanical neck pain and cervicogenic headache. Neurosurgery. 2007;60(1 Suppl 1):S21–7 [Review].
9. Binder AI. Cervical spondylosis and neck pain. BMJ. 2007;334(7592):527–31 [Review].
10. Bykowski JL, Wong WH. Role of facet joints in spine pain and image-guided treatment: a review. AJNR Am J Neuroradiol. 2012;33(8):1419–26 [Review].

11. Falco FJ, Datta S, Manchikanti L, Sehgal N, Geffert S, Singh V, et al. An updated review of the diagnostic utility of cervical facet joint injections. Pain Physician. 2012;15(6):E807–38 [Review].
12. Gerwin RD. Diagnosis of myofascial pain syndrome. Phys Med Rehabil Clin N Am. 2014;25(2):341–55 [Review].
13. Manchikanti L, Dunbar EE, Wargo BW, Shah RV, Derby R, Cohen SP. Systematic review of cervical discography as a diagnostic test for chronic spinal pain. Pain Physician. 2009; 12(2):305–21 [Review].
14. Oberstein EM, Carpintero M, Hopkins A. Neck pain from a rheumatologic perspective. Phys Med Rehabil Clin N Am. 2011;22(3):485–502, ix [Review].
15. Polston DW. Cervical radiculopathy. Neurol Clin. 2007;25(2):373–85 [Review].
16. Van Zundert J, Huntoon M, Patijn J, Lataster A, Mekhail N, van Kleef M, et al. 4. Cervical radicular pain. Pain Pract. 2010;10(1):1–17 [Case Reports Review].
17. Malanga GA. The diagnosis and treatment of cervical radiculopathy. Med Sci Sports Exerc. 1997;29 Suppl 7:S236–45.
18. Litchy WJ, O'Fallon WM, Kurland LT. Epidemiology of cervical radiculopathy. A population-based study from Rochester, Minnesota, 1976 through 1990. Brain. 1994;117(Pt 2):325–35 [Research Support, U.S. Gov't, P.H.S.].
19. Wilbourn AJ, Aminoff MJ. AAEE minimonograph #32: the electrophysiologic examination in patients with radiculopathies. Muscle Nerve. 1988;11(11):1099–114.
20. Henderson CM, Hennessy RG, Shuey Jr HM, Shackelford EG. Posterior-lateral foraminotomy as an exclusive operative technique for cervical radiculopathy: a review of 846 consecutively operated cases. Neurosurgery. 1983;13(5):504–12.
21. Nordin M, Carragee EJ, Hogg-Johnson S, Weiner SS, Hurwitz EL, Peloso PM, et al. Assessment of neck pain and its associated disorders: results of the Bone and Joint Decade 2000–2010 Task Force on Neck Pain and Its Associated Disorders. Spine (Phila Pa 1976). 2008;33 Suppl 4:S101–22.
22. Wainner RS, Fritz JM, Irrgang JJ, Boninger ML, Delitto A, Allison S. Reliability and diagnostic accuracy of the clinical examination and patient self-report measures for cervical radiculopathy. Spine (Phila Pa 1976). 2003;28(1):52–62.
23. Sandmark H, Nisell R. Validity of five common manual neck pain provoking tests. Scand J Rehabil Med. 1995;27(3):131–6.
24. Matsumoto M, Fujimura Y, Suzuki N, Yoshiaki T, Shiga H. Cervical curvature in acute whiplash injuries: prospective comparative study with asymptomatic subjects. Injury. 1998;29(10):775–8.
25. Boden SD, McCowin PR, Davis DO, Dina TS, Mark AS, Wiesel S. Abnormal magnetic-resonance scans of the cervical spine in asymptomatic subjects. A prospective investigation. J Bone Joint Surg Am. 1990;72(8):1178–84.
26. Teresi LM, Lufkin RB, Reicher MA, Moffit BJ, Vinuela FV, Wilson GM, et al. Asymptomatic degenerative disk disease and spondylosis of the cervical spine: MR imaging. Radiology. 1987;164(1):83–8.
27. Carette S, Fehlings MG. Clinical practice. Cervical radiculopathy. N Engl J Med. 2005;353(4):392–9 [Review].
28. Nardin RA, Patel MR, Gudas TF, Rutkove SB, Raynor EM. Electromyography and magnetic resonance imaging in the evaluation of radiculopathy. Muscle Nerve. 1999;22(2):151–5 [Comparative Study].
29. Dwyer A, Aprill C, Bogduk N. Cervical zygapophyseal joint pain patterns. I: A study in normal volunteers. Spine (Phila Pa 1976). 1990;15(6):453–7.
30. Manchikanti L, Boswell MV, Singh V, Pampati V, Damron KS, Beyer CD. Prevalence of facet joint pain in chronic spinal pain of cervical, thoracic, and lumbar regions. BMC Musculoskelet Disord. 2004;5:15.
31. Manchikanti L, Singh V, Rivera J, Pampati V. Prevalence of cervical facet joint pain in chronic neck pain. Pain Physician. 2002;5(3):243–9.

32. Speldewinde GC, Bashford GM, Davidson IR. Diagnostic cervical zygapophyseal joint blocks for chronic cervical pain. Med J Aust. 2001;174(4):174–6.
33. Yin W, Bogduk N. The nature of neck pain in a private pain clinic in the United States. Pain Med. 2008;9(2):196–203.
34. Barnsley L, Lord SM, Wallis BJ, Bogduk N. The prevalence of chronic cervical zygapophysial joint pain after whiplash. Spine (Phila Pa 1976). 1995;20(1):20–5. discussion 6. [Research Support, Non-U.S. Gov't].
35. Lord SM, Barnsley L, Wallis BJ, Bogduk N. Chronic cervical zygapophysial joint pain after whiplash. A placebo-controlled prevalence study. Spine (Phila Pa 1976). 1996;21(15):1737–44. discussion 44–5. [Clinical Trial Randomized Controlled Trial Research Support, Non-U.S. Gov't].
36. van Eerd M, Patijn J, Lataster A, Rosenquist RW, van Kleef M, Mekhail N, et al. 5. Cervical facet pain. Pain Pract. 2010;10(2):113–23 [Review].
37. Cooper G, Bailey B, Bogduk N. Cervical zygapophysial joint pain maps. Pain Med. 2007;8(4):344–53.
38. Yang H, Haldeman S, Nakata A, Choi B, Delp L, Baker D. Work-related risk factors for neck pain in the US working population. Spine (Phila Pa 1976). 2015;40(3):184–92.
39. Hallman DM, Gupta N, Mathiassen SE, Holtermann A. Association between objectively measured sitting time and neck-shoulder pain among blue-collar workers. Int Arch Occup Environ Health. 2015;88(8):1031–42.
40. Cohen SP, Bajwa ZH, Kraemer JJ, Dragovich A, Williams KA, Stream J, et al. Factors predicting success and failure for cervical facet radiofrequency denervation: a multi-center analysis. Reg Anesth Pain Med. 2007;32(6):495–503.
41. van der Donk J, Schouten JS, Passchier J, van Romunde LK, Valkenburg HA. The associations of neck pain with radiological abnormalities of the cervical spine and personality traits in a general population. J Rheumatol. 1991;18(12):1884–9 [Research Support, Non-U.S. Gov't].
42. Lord SM, Barnsley L, Wallis BJ, McDonald GJ, Bogduk N. Percutaneous radio-frequency neurotomy for chronic cervical zygapophyseal-joint pain. N Engl J Med. 1996;335(23):1721–6 [Clinical Trial Randomized Controlled Trial Research Support, Non-U.S. Gov't].
43. Bogduk N. Medical management of acute cervical radicular pain: an evidence-based approach. 1st ed. Newcastle, N.S.W.: Newcastle Bone and Joint Institute, Royal Newcastle Hospital; 1999.
44. Groen GJ, Baljet B, Drukker J. Nerves and nerve plexuses of the human vertebral column. Am J Anat. 1990;188(3):282–96.
45. Bogduk N, International Spine Intervention Society. Standards Committee. Practice guidelines for spinal diagnostic and treatment procedures. 1st ed. San Francisco: International Spine Intervention Society; 2004.
46. Schellhas KP, Smith MD, Gundry CR, Pollei SR. Cervical discogenic pain. Prospective correlation of magnetic resonance imaging and discography in asymptomatic subjects and pain sufferers. Spine (Phila Pa 1976). 1996;21(3):300–11; discussion 11–2.
47. Parfenchuck TAMD, Janssen MEDO. A correlation of cervical magnetic resonance imaging and discography/computed tomographic discograms. Spine (Phila Pa 1976). 1994; 19(24):2819–23.
48. Bogduk N, Aprill C. On the nature of neck pain, discography and cervical zygapophysial joint blocks. Pain. 1993;54(2):213–7.
49. Fricton JR, Kroening R, Haley D, Siegert R. Myofascial pain syndrome of the head and neck: a review of clinical characteristics of 164 patients. Oral Surg Oral Med Oral Pathol. 1985;60(6):615–23.
50. Bennett R. Myofascial pain syndromes and their evaluation. Best Pract Res Clin Rheumatol. 2007;21(3):427–45 [Review].
51. Yap EC. Myofascial pain—an overview. Ann Acad Med Singapore. 2007;36(1):43–8 [Review].

52. Kasch H, Qerama E, Kongsted A, Bach FW, Bendix T, Jensen TS. Deep muscle pain, tender points and recovery in acute whiplash patients: a 1-year follow-up study. Pain. 2008;140(1):65–73 [Research Support, Non-U.S. Gov't].

53. Gerwin RD. A review of myofascial pain and fibromyalgia—factors that promote their persistence. Acupunct Med. 2005;23(3):121–34 [Review].

54. Ekbom K, Torhall J, Annell K, Traff J. Magnetic resonance imaging in retropharyngeal tendinitis. Cephalalgia. 1994;14(4):266–9; discussion 57.

55. Cha TD, An HS. Cervical spine manifestations in patients with inflammatory arthritides. Nat Rev Rheumatol. 2013;9(7):423–32 [Review].

56. Rawlins BA, Girardi FP, Boachie-Adjei O. Rheumatoid arthritis of the cervical spine. Rheum Dis Clin North Am. 1998;24(1):55–65.

57. Reiter MF, Boden SD. Inflammatory disorders of the cervical spine. Spine (Phila Pa 1976). 1998;23(24):2755–66.

58. Ramos-Remus C, Gomez-Vargas A, Guzman-Guzman JL, Jimenez-Gil F, Gamez-Nava JI, Gonzalez-Lopez L, et al. Frequency of atlantoaxial subluxation and neurologic involvement in patients with ankylosing spondylitis. J Rheumatol. 1995;22(11):2120–5 [Research Support, Non-U.S. Gov't].

59. Takahashi M, Yamashita Y, Sakamoto Y, Kojima R. Chronic cervical cord compression: clinical significance of increased signal intensity on MR images. Radiology. 1989;173(1):219–24.

60. Riew KD, Hilibrand AS, Palumbo MA, Sethi N, Bohlman HH. Diagnosing basilar invagination in the rheumatoid patient. The reliability of radiographic criteria. J Bone Joint Surg Am. 2001;83-A(2):194–200.

61. Manchikanti L, Falco FJ, Diwan S, Hirsch JA, Smith HS. Cervical radicular pain: the role of interlaminar and transforaminal epidural injections. Curr Pain Headache Rep. 2014;18(1):389 [Review].

62. Niemisto L, Kalso E, Malmivaara A, Seitsalo S, Hurri H. Radiofrequency denervation for neck and back pain: a systematic review within the framework of the cochrane collaboration back review group. Spine (Phila Pa 1976). 2003;28(16):1877–88 [Meta-Analysis Review].

63. Deer TR, Skaribas IM, Haider N, Salmon J, Kim C, Nelson C, et al. Effectiveness of cervical spinal cord stimulation for the management of chronic pain. Neuromodulation. 2014;17(3):265–71. discussion 71. [Evaluation Studies Multicenter Study Review].

64. Deer TR. Polyanalgesic consensus conference 2012. Neuromodulation. 2012;15(5):418–9 [Consensus Development Conference].

Chapter 5
Revision Surgery and Alternative Treatment Options for Recurrent Pain Following Spinal Surgery

Aleka Scoco, Jonathan P. Miller, and Jennifer A. Sweet

Key Points

- Many patients who undergo spinal surgery have continued postoperative neuropathic and/or back pain.
- The persistence of pain following spinal surgery may represent the development of new or recurrent pathology, which may require revision surgery.
- Neuromodulation may be an alternative option for patients with unrelieved pain after previous spinal surgery.
- Spinal cord stimulation demonstrates superiority to repeat spinal surgery in select patients.

Introduction

Low back pain (LBP) accounts for the second most common pathology resulting in disability in the USA [1], and there has yet to be a standard treatment algorithm for the management of such patients. Over the last century, extensive research has been

A. Scoco, B.A.
Case Western Reserve University School of Medicine,
2109 Adelbert Rd, Cleveland, OH 44106, USA
e-mail: ans98@case.edu

J.P. Miller, M.D., F.A.A.N.S., F.A.C.S. • J.A. Sweet, M.D. (✉)
Functional and Restorative Neurosurgery Center, University Hospital Case Medical Center,
11100 Euclid Ave., Mailstop 5042, Cleveland, OH 44106, USA

Neurological Surgery, Case Western Reserve University School of Medicine,
11100 Euclid Ave., Mailstop 5042, Cleveland, OH 44106, USA
e-mail: Jonathan.Miller@uhhospitals.org; jennifer.sweet@uhhospitals.org

© Springer International Publishing Switzerland 2016
S.M. Falowski, J.E. Pope (eds.), *Integrating Pain Treatment into Your Spine Practice*, DOI 10.1007/978-3-319-27796-7_5

done investigating surgical treatment options for patients suffering from such pain, reflected by the rising surgery rates of novel, complex spinal fusions [2]. In the USA alone, there was a 15-fold increase in the rate of complex spinal fusion procedures for back pain from 2003 to 2007 [1]. However, complication rates for complex surgeries are much higher than for simpler procedures [2]. In addition, the sequelae from such procedures can result in epidural scarring, which may produce persistent LBP and neuropathic extremity pain, resulting in overall functional impairment [2]. This scenario can be frustrating to both physicians and patients alike, as a clear management strategy is often lacking. Thus the goal of this chapter is to identify indications for revision spine surgery versus alternative pain management options for patients with chronic neuropathic pain and LBP after prior lumbar surgery.

Identification

The primary indications for surgical intervention for degenerative spine disease include compression of neural elements and/or structural instability, either of which can result in LBP and lower extremity radicular pain. For the right patients, surgical interventions can result in substantial improvement in overall pain and quality of life [3, 4]. However, for patients who have already undergone surgery, indications for subsequent treatment options, including surgical revision, are less clear.

Revision Spinal Surgery Versus Alternative Treatment Options for Postoperative Pain

The persistence of pain following surgery of the spine may represent the development of new or recurrent pathology, such as re-herniation of a disc, persistent stenosis, instability, or pseudoarthrosis, all of which may be indications for revision surgery [5–8]. A careful history and physical examination can help to determine the etiology of a patient's postoperative pain. For example, mechanical back pain after a short period of post-surgical pain relief can be indicative of pseudoarthrosis or instability [5], and dynamic X-rays or a CT scan may help to demonstrate such findings. Similarly, if a patient has complaints and neurological findings concerning enough to warrant postoperative imaging, an MRI may demonstrate re-herniation of a disc or other structural abnormalities. Such findings may also necessitate revision surgery.

However, the challenges in management arise in situations in which neuropathic lower extremity pain and persistent LBP are present without impressive findings on imaging. Whether or not these symptoms exist from epidural fibrosis [2] or an overall progression of the degenerative process which led to the initial surgery remains unclear, as does the association between the degree of fibrosis on MRI and clinical

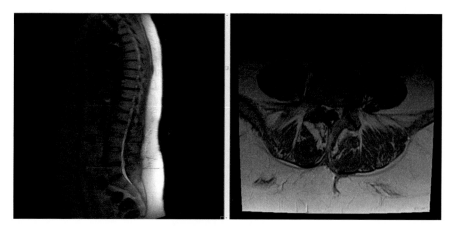

Fig. 5.1 Sagittal (*left*) and axial (*right*) MRI demonstrating epidural fibrosis surrounding the left nerve root in a patient with persistent postoperative neuropathic lower extremity pain and low back pain

outcome [9]. An example of postoperative scar tissue surrounding a nerve root is demonstrated in Fig. 5.1. Ultimately, roughly 30 % of patients who undergo spine surgery for purposes of pain alleviation still fail to improve postoperatively [10, 11]. This raises the question of what to do with patients who fail surgery or present with recurrent symptoms. The physical, emotional, and economical costs of failed pain relief with prior spinal surgery places a significant burden on both patients and society.

Failed Back Surgery Syndrome

For patients in whom there is persistent neuropathic and LBP following surgery, with evidence of fibrosis or otherwise unremarkable findings on MRI, alternative options to revision surgery are warranted. The most supported indication for these treatments is failed back surgery syndrome (FBSS). This includes patients with chronic back pain and neuropathic lower extremity pain following spinal surgery, often in the setting of normal post-operative imaging [12]. In situations of FBSS, revision spinal surgeries have been shown to result in improvement in only 20–30 % of patients [13, 14]. In fact, data has suggested that patients with persistent chronic LBP with a neuropathic component, may not be easily correctable with revision surgery [15, 16].

The term "failed back surgery syndrome" may be a misnomer, given the diverse profile of risk factors and uncertain pathophysiology of the disease [1]. In addition to common postoperative conditions such as recurrent disc herniation, fibrosis-associated neuropathic pain, degenerative changes, facet joint pain, arachnoiditis, and pseudoarthrosis, other known associated risk factors for FBSS include age, smoking, obesity, lack of physical exercise, deconditioning, and depression [17–19]. The presence of these conditions affirms the need to control comorbidities.

Patients with FBSS are thought to develop epidural fibrosis following surgery due to postoperative inflammation, tissue manipulation, or bleeding into the epidural space. The scar tissue may then result in nerve entrapment, reduced tissue perfusion, or functional abnormalities in the subarachnoid space [20]. The impact of this fibrosis in postsurgical patients has been strongly associated with persistent LBP [21]. However, studies show no clinical correlation between the degree of fibrosis on MRI and clinical outcome [9]. Moreover, repeat surgery for epidural fibrosis has not been associated with improvement of pain [22].

Evidence

Conservative Treatment Options

First-line treatment options for patients with post-operative chronic back and radicular pain without significant radiographic findings traditionally consists of conservative management options [23, 24]. Such treatment strategies include exercise therapy with a supervised physical therapist, multidisciplinary bio-psychosocial rehabilitation, and medical treatment with opioid and non-narcotic medications. There is also evidence supporting the use of alternative medicine treatments such as acupuncture, yoga, thermal modalities, and acupressure [24–26]. Providers must tailor therapy to individual patients and be cautious in selecting specific treatments as well as promising results.

Steroid injections may also be indicated to alleviate both back and neuropathic pain by reducing inflammation. There are numerous types of injections such as interlaminar, transforaminal, and caudal approaches, which may all play a role in the treatment of symptoms, prior to or instead of surgery [20, 21]. Benefit may be achieved through a series of three injections over a 6–12 month period, for longer-lasting pain relief. The drawbacks of steroid injections are the often short duration of pain control, as well as the immunosuppressive properties of steroid use.

Neuromodulation

The use of neuromodulation has become increasingly popular for the treatment of chronic LBP and radicular pain following spinal surgery that has failed conservative measures, and may be a better option than repeat spine surgery. Neuromodulation consists of the implementation of technologies that act on neural structures, often via the delivery of electrical stimulation or pharmacological agents, to restore

Table 5.1 PROCESS trial outcomes summary

Treatment	Number of patients	% Achieving primary outcome (at 6 months)	% Achieving primary outcome (at 24 months)
Spinal cord stimulation (SCS)	50	48 % ($p=0.001$)	37 % ($p=0.003$)
Conservative medical management (CMM)	43	9 % ($p=0.001$)	2 % ($p=0.003$)

function and/or influence symptoms of disease. Examples of neuromodulation for the management of patients with persistent neuropathic lower extremity pain and LBP following spinal surgery include spinal cord stimulation (SCS) and intrathecal pain pumps (ITP).

Spinal Cord Stimulation (SCS)

SCS offers a promising treatment option to patients with persistent postoperative neuropathic pain. When Melzack and Wall published their iconic paper on gate control theory in 1965, and Norman Shealy first discovered the potential therapeutic value of SCS, so began a revolution in the way pain management is achieved [27, 28]. Though evidence for the efficacy of SCS for patients with FBSS was established in the 1990s, its mechanism of action and optimization are still being explored, with current research focusing on the delivery of new stimulation parameters [29]. Despite the many unknowns associated with SCS, the use of SCS for the treatment of patients with chronic back and neuropathic pain has gained popularity, and has even proven to be cost effective for health care as well [30]. Currently, the annual number of stimulators implanted is increasing, and has become critical in the armamentarium of clinicians treating such patients [31, 32].

Multiple studies have demonstrated significant improvements in neuropathic extremity pain, with or without back pain in a majority of patients with few complications [33, 34]. In one of the first large series of SCS for FBSS, patients were treated with SCS and followed for 4 years [35]. Overall, patients reported more than 60 % subjective improvement of pain, a significant reduction in medication usage, and an increased working capacity [36]. A study by North et al. also demonstrated the efficacy of SCS for FBSS [37]. The authors found a successful outcome, defined as at least 50 % sustained relief of pain and patient satisfaction, in a majority of 50 FBSS patients after SCS implantation. A subsequent study of 153 patients with FBSS had similar findings, with 52 % of patients achieving pain relief after SCS with an average follow-up period of 7 years [35]. In a large multicenter study, the PROCESS trial, SCS was compared to conservative medical management [38–40]. The results were impressive, showing the superiority of SCS treatment over CMM; specific outcome data can be seen in Table 5.1. Several other investigators have since affirmed SCS efficacy with respect to improvements in functional capacity in addition to pain [41–45]. As such, various American and international regulatory

Table 5.2 International consensus and guidelines

Society	Recommendation for SCS use for FBSS
American College of Occupational and Environmental Medicine (ACOEM) (based on recently revised data [46]	Strong evidence for the use of SCS for FBSS
American Society of Interventional Pain Physicians [32]	Strong recommendations for the short term and moderate strength for prolonged use
British Pain Society [47]	Recommended treatment for neuropathic pain
Canadian Pain Society [48]	Grade B strength recommendation
Cochrane review based on Agency for Healthcare Research and Quality (AHRQ) criteria [49]	Level II-1 or II-2 evidence for relieving intractable pain of FBSS on a long-term basis
European Federation of Neurological Societies (EFNS) [50]	Level II evidence

and pain societies have confirmed the role of SCS for the treatment of FBSS. A summary of these recommendations can be found in Table 5.2. Even when compared to other treatment options such as repeat spinal surgery which can carry an improvement of 20–30 %, there are few modalities that can carry such success as SCS.

In order to optimize the efficacy of SCS treatment for patients suffering from FBSS, these patients need to meet certain selection criteria [32]. Up to 36–40 % post-SCS implant patients still have ongoing disability and pain, underscoring the need for stringent inclusion and exclusion criteria [51]. As with any intervention, patient selection is crucial. To qualify for an SCS treatment trial for chronic LBP and lower extremity radicular pain, patients need to have failed at least 3–6 months of adequate conservative medical management. This includes physical therapy, analgesics, both opioid and nonopioid, and epidural steroid injections. Completion of a pain psychology evaluation is typically advised prior to SCS, and for placement of paddle SCS leads, thoracic imaging is recommended to ensure sufficient space for the lead without causing spinal cord compression. Furthermore, a completed successful SCS trial, defined as ≥50 % pain relief prior to permanent stimulator and lead implant is essential to ensure efficacy of the treatment [52]. Patients with a positive SCS trial have increased success post-implantation when compared to those who fail to respond [53].

However, as with any surgery, SCS may have complications. In the PROCESS trial, 19 (45 %) of the 42 patients still receiving SCS at 24-months experienced a total of 34 SCS-related complications, primarily related to hardware migration and biological events including wound breakdown or pain at the incision site [40]. Only a small proportion of events (15 %) were attributed to loss of therapeutic effect.

SCS Versus Revision Therapy for FBSS

When directly comparing SCS versus reoperation for treatment of FBSS, there is clear superiority of SCS treatment [51]. In 2005, North et al. published a randomized control trial to investigate the issue of surgical revision; he randomly assigned patients with FBSS to receive either SCS or reoperation. SCS was more successful than reoperation (9 of 19 patients vs. 3 of 26 patients, $p < 0.01$), and patients initially randomized to SCS were significantly less likely to cross over than were those randomized to reoperation (5 of 24 patients vs. 14 of 26 patients, $p < 0.02$) [51].

There is also evidence to suggest that the sooner a diagnosis of FBSS can be recognized and subsequently treated with SCS, the better the prognosis for treatment efficacy [54]. SCS performed early in the course of a patient's chronic pain process is associated with better outcomes than SCS performed late in the disease [52].

Intrathecal Pain Pumps

Intrathecal pain pumps function by delivering programmable doses of drugs, such as an opioid alone or in combination with a local anesthetic agent, directly to the cerebrospinal fluid. At present approved labeling is for either Morphine or Ziconatide to be delivered via an intrathecal therapy. Although the efficacy of intrathecal pain pumps for the treatment of FBSS has yet to be demonstrated in a large-scale randomized clinical trial [55], there is evidence supporting the use of implantable intrathecal infusion systems for FBSS for both short-term and long-term relief of symptoms, particularly for the nociceptive back pain component [56]. Similar to SCS, patients are encouraged to undergo a successful trial prior to initiation of therapy.

Summary

Persistent postoperative lower extremity neuropathic pain and low back pain following spinal surgery affects a large number of patients. While revision surgery may be indicated in cases of a new or recurrent pathology as confirmed on history, physical, and imaging evaluations, many patients are not candidates for reoperations. As such, an understanding of the pathophysiology of their symptoms, as well as the currently available alternative treatment options, is essential. This includes physical therapy, multidisciplinary rehabilitation, and pain management strategies as well as neuromodulation techniques, such as spinal cord stimulation and intrathecal pain pumps.

References

1. Amirdelfan K, McRoberts P, Deer TR. The differential diagnosis of low back pain: a primer on the evolving paradigm. Neuromodulation Technol Neural Interface [Internet]. 2014;17:11–7. doi:10.1111/ner.12173.
2. Deyo RA, Mirza SK, Martin BI, Kreuter W, Goodman DC, Jarvik JG. Trends, major medical complications, and charges associated with surgery for lumbar spinal stenosis in older adults. JAMA. 2010;303:1259–65.
3. Weinstein JN, Tosteson TD, Lurie JD, Tosteson AN, Hanscom B, Skinner JS, et al. Surgical vs nonoperative treatment for lumbar disk herniation: the Spine Patient Outcomes Research Trial (SPORT): a randomized trial. JAMA. 2006;296:2441–50.
4. Weinstein JN, Lurie JD, Tosteson TD, Zhao W, Blood EA, Tosteson ANA, et al. Surgical compared with nonoperative treatment for lumbar degenerative spondylolisthesis. Four-year results in the Spine Patient Outcomes Research Trial (SPORT) randomized and observational cohorts. J Bone Joint Surg Am [Internet]. 2009 [cited 2015 May 23];91:1295–304. Available from: http://www.pubmedcentral.nih.gov/articlerender.fcgi?artid=2686131&tool=pmcentrez&rendertype=abstract.
5. Elgafy H, Vaccaro AR, Chapman JR, Dvorak MF. Rationale of revision lumbar spine surgery. Glob Spine J [Internet]. 2012 [cited 2015 May 23];2:7–14. Available from: http://www.pubmedcentral.nih.gov/articlerender.fcgi?artid=3864481&tool=pmcentrez&rendertype=abstract.
6. McAnany SJ, Baird EO, Overley SC, Kim JS, Qureshi SA, Anderson PA. A meta-analysis of the clinical and fusion results following treatment of symptomatic cervical pseudarthrosis. Glob Spine J [Internet]. 2015 [cited 2015 May 23];5:148–55. Available from: http://www.pubmedcentral.nih.gov/articlerender.fcgi?artid=4369200&tool=pmcentrez&rendertype=abstract.
7. Kostuik JP. Complications and surgical revision for failed disc arthroplasty. Spine J [Internet]. 2004 [cited 2015 May 23];4:289S–291S. Available from: http://www.sciencedirect.com/science/article/pii/S1529943004005868.
8. Koerner JD, Kepler CK, Albert TJ. Revision surgery for failed cervical spine reconstruction: review article. HSS J [Internet]. 2015 [cited 2015 May 23];11:2–8. Available from: http://www.ncbi.nlm.nih.gov/pubmed/25737662.
9. Almeida DB, Prandini MN, Awamura Y, Vitola ML, Simião MP, Milano JB, et al. Outcome following lumbar disc surgery: the role of fibrosis. Acta Neurochir (Wien) [Internet]. 2008 [cited 2015 Mar 26];150:1167–76. Available from: http://www.ncbi.nlm.nih.gov/pubmed/18936878.
10. Segal R, Stacey BR, Rudy TE, Baser S, Markham J. Spinal cord stimulation revisited. Neurol Res. 1998;20(5):391–6.
11. North RB, Ewend MG, Lawton MT, Piantadosi S. Spinal cord stimulation for chronic, intractable pain: superiority of "multi-channel" devices. Pain. 1991;44:119–30.
12. Van Buyten JP, Linderoth B. "The failed back surgery syndrome": definition and therapeutic algorithms—an update. Eur J Pain Suppl [Internet]. European Federation of International Association for the Study of Pain Chapters; 2010;4:273–86. doi:10.1016/j.eujps.2010.09.006.
13. North RB, Campbell JN, James CS, Conover-Walker MK, Wang H, Piantadosi S, et al. Failed back surgery syndrome: 5-year follow-up in 102 patients undergoing repeated operation. Neurosurgery [Internet]. 1991 [cited 2015 Mar 26];28:685–90; discussion 690–1. Available from: http://www.ncbi.nlm.nih.gov/pubmed/1831546.
14. Fritsch EW, Heisel J, Rupp S. The failed back surgery syndrome: reasons, intraoperative findings, and long-term results: a report of 182 operative treatments. Spine (Phila Pa 1976). 1996;21:626–33.
15. Vaccaro AR, Silber JS. Post-traumatic spinal deformity. Spine (Phila Pa 1976). 2001;26:111–8.
16. Onesti ST. Failed back syndrome. Neurologist [Internet]. 2004 [cited 2015 Mar 26];10:259–64. Available from: http://www.ncbi.nlm.nih.gov/pubmed/15335443.

17. Chan C, Peng P. Failed back surgery syndrome. Pain Med. 2011;12:577–606.
18. Rodrigues FF, Dozza DC, De Oliveira CR, De Castro RG. Failed back surgery syndrome: casuistic and etiology. Arq Neuropsiquiatr. 2006;64:757–61.
19. Skaf G, Bouclaous C, Alaraj A, Chamoun R. Clinical outcome of surgical treatment of failed back surgery syndrome. Surg Neurol. 2005;64:483–8.
20. Veizi E, Hayek S. Interventional therapies for chronic low back pain. Neuromodulation Technol Neural Interface [Internet]. 2014;17:31–45. doi:10.1111/ner.12250.
21. Long DM. Chronic adhesive spinal arachnoiditis: pathogenesis, prognosis, and treatment. Neurosurg Q [Internet]. 1992;2. Available from: http://journals.lww.com/neurosurgery-quarterly/Fulltext/1992/12000/Chronic_Adhesive_Spinal_Arachnoiditis_.4.aspx.
22. Ohnmeiss DD, Rashbaum RF. Patient satisfaction with spinal cord stimulation for predominant complaints of chronic, intractable low back pain. Spine J. 2001;1:358–63.
23. Van Buyten J-P, Al-Kaisy A, Smet I, Palmisani S, Smith T. High-frequency spinal cord stimulation for the treatment of chronic back pain patients: results of a prospective multicenter European clinical study. Neuromodulation [Internet]. 2012;16:59–65; discussion 65–6. Available from: http://www.ncbi.nlm.nih.gov/pubmed/23199157.
24. Wellington J. Noninvasive and alternative management of chronic low back pain (efficacy and outcomes). Neuromodulation Technol Neural Interface [Internet]. 2014;17:24–30. doi:10.1111/ner.12078.
25. Furlan AD, van Tulder MW, Cherkin DC, Tsukayama H, Lao L, Koes BW, et al. Acupuncture and dry-needling for low back pain. Cochrane Database Syst Rev. 2005;CD001351.
26. Manheimer E, White A, Berman B, Forys K, Ernst E. Meta-analysis: acupuncture for low back pain. Ann Intern Med [Internet]. 2005 [cited 2015 Feb 21];142:651–63. Available from: http://www.ncbi.nlm.nih.gov/pubmed/15838072.
27. Melzack R, Wall PD. Pain mechanisms: a new theory. Science. 1965;150:971–9.
28. Shealy CN, Mortimer JT, Reswick JB. Electrical inhibition of pain by stimulation of the dorsal columns: preliminary clinical report. Anesth Analg. 1967;46:489–91.
29. Deer TR, Thomson S, Pope JE, Russo M, Luscombe F, Levy R. International neuromodulation society critical assessment: guideline review of implantable neurostimulation devices. Neuromodulation [Internet]. 2014;2014:678–85. Available from: http://www.ncbi.nlm.nih.gov/pubmed/24802237.
30. Deer T, Skaribas I, Nelson C, Tracy J, Meloy S, Darnule A, et al. Interim results from the partnership for advancement in neuromodulation pain registry. Neuromodulation Technol Neural Interface [Internet]. 2013;17:656–64. doi:10.1111/ner.12154.
31. Manchikanti L, Singh V, Pampati V, Smith HS, Hirsch JA. Analysis of growth of interventional techniques in managing chronic pain in the Medicare population: a 10-year evaluation from 1997 to 2006. Pain Physician. 2009;12:9–34.
32. Deer T, Pope J, Hayek S, Narouze S, Patil P, Foreman R, et al. Neurostimulation for the treatment of axial back pain: a review of mechanisms, techniques, outcomes, and future advances. Neuromodulation Technol Neural Interface [Internet]. 2014;17:52–68. doi:10.1111/j.1525-1403.2012.00530.x.
33. Burchiel KJ, Anderson VC, Brown FD, Fessler RG, Friedman WA, Pelofsky S, et al. Prospective, multicenter study of spinal cord stimulation for relierf of chronic back and extremity pain. Spine (Phila Pa 1976). 1996;21(23):2786–94.
34. Ohnmeiss DD, Rashbaum RF, Bogdanffy GM. Prospective outcome evaluation of spinal cord stimulation in patients with intractable leg pain. Spine (Phila Pa 1976). 1996;21(11):1344–50.
35. North RB, Kidd DH, Zahurak M, James CS, Long DM, Burchiel KJ, et al. Spinal cord stimulation for chronic, intractable pain: experience over two decades. Neurosurgery [Internet]. 1993;32:384–95. Available from: http://ovidsp.ovid.com/ovidweb.cgi?T=JS&CSC=Y&NEWS=N&PAGE=fulltext&AN=00006123-199303000-00008&D=ovft&PDF=y.
36. De la Porte C, Siegfried J. Lumbosacral spinal fibrosis (spinal arachnoiditis). Its diagnosis and treatment by spinal cord stimulation. Spine (Phila Pa 1976). 1983;8:593–603.

37. North RB, Ewend MG, Lawton MT, Kidd DH, Piantadosi S. Failed back surgery syndrome: 5-year follow-up after spinal cord stimulator implantation. Neurosurgery. 1991;28:692–9.
38. Kumar K, North R, Taylor R, Sculpher M, Van den Abeele C, Gehring M, et al. Spinal cord stimulation vs. conventional medical management: a prospective, randomized, controlled, multicenter study of patients with failed back surgery syndrome (PROCESS study). Neuromodulation [Internet]. 2005;8:213–8. Available from: http://www.ncbi.nlm.nih.gov/pubmed/22151547.
39. Kumar K, Taylor RS, Jacques L, Eldabe S, Meglio M, Molet J, et al. Spinal cord stimulation versus conventional medical management for neuropathic pain: a multicentre randomised controlled trial in patients with failed back surgery syndrome. Pain. 2007;132:179–88.
40. Kumar K, Taylor RS, Jacques L, Eldabe S, Meglio M, Molet J, et al. The effects of spinal cord stimulation in neuropathic pain are sustained: a 24-month follow-up of the prospective randomized controlled multicenter trial of the effectiveness of spinal cord stimulation. Neurosurgery. 2008;63:762–8.
41. Kumar K, Toth C. The role of spinal cord stimulation in the treatment of chronic pain postlaminectomy. Curr Rev Pain. 1998;2:85–92.
42. Van Buyten JP, Van Zundert J, Milbouw G. Treatment of failed back surgery syndrome patients with low back and leg pain: a pilot study of a new dual lead spinal cord stimulation system. Neuromodulation [Internet]. 1999;2:258–65. Available from: http://www.ncbi.nlm.nih.gov/pubmed/22151259.
43. Barolat G, Oakley JC, Law JD, North RB, Ketcik B, Sharan A. Epidural spinal cord stimulation with a multiple electrode paddle lead is effective in treating intractable low back pain. Neuromodulation. 2001;4:59–66.
44. Leveque J-C, Villavicencio AT, Bulsara KR, Rubin L, et al. Spinal cord stimulation for failed back surgery syndrome [Internet]. Neuromodulation Technol Neural Interface. 2001 [cited 2015 Mar 26]. p. 1–9. Available from: http://journals.ohiolink.edu/ejc/article.cgi?issn=1094715 9&issue=v04i0001&article=1_scsffbss.
45. Kumar K, Wilson JR, Taylor RS, Gupta S. Complications of spinal cord stimulation, suggestions to improve outcome, and financial impact. J Neurosurg Spine. 2006;5:191–203.
46. Manchikanti L, Singh V, Derby R, Schultz DM, Benyamin RM, Prager JP, et al. Reassessment of evidence synthesis of occupational medicine practice guidelines for interventional pain management. Pain Physician [Internet]. 2008;11:393–482. Available from: http://www.ncbi.nlm.nih.gov/pubmed/18690276.
47. Collett B, Collins D, Eldridge P, et al. Spinal Cord Stimulation for the management of pain: recommendations for best clinical practice. In: Simpson KR, Stannard C, Raphael J, editors. A consensus document prepared on behalf of the British Pain Society in consultation with the Society of British Neurological Surgeons. London: The British Pain Society; 2009.
48. Mailis A, Taenzer P. Evidence-based guideline for neuropathic pain interventional treatments: spinal cord stimulation, intravenous infusions, epidural injections and nerve blocks. Pain Res Manag [Internet]. 2012 [cited 2015 Feb 25];17:150–8. Available from: http://www.pubmedcentral.nih.gov/articlerender.fcgi?artid=3401085&tool=pmcentrez&rendertype=abstract.
49. Frey ME, Manchikanti L, Benyamin RM, Schultz DM, Smith HS, Cohen SP. Spinal cord stimulation for patients with failed back surgery syndrome: a systematic review. Pain Physician [Internet]. 2009;12:379–97. Available from: http://www.ncbi.nlm.nih.gov/pubmed/19305486.
50. Airaksinen O, Herno A, Turunen V, Saari T, Suomlainen O. Surgical outcome of 438 patients treated surgically for lumbar spinal stenosis. Spine (Phila Pa 1976) [Internet]. 1997 [cited 2015 Mar 26];22:2278–82. Available from: http://www.ncbi.nlm.nih.gov/pubmed/9346149.
51. Eldabe S, Kumar K, Buchser E, Taylor RS. An analysis of the components of pain, function, and health-related quality of life in patients with failed back surgery syndrome treated with spinal cord stimulation or conventional medical management. Neuromodulation. 2010;13:201–9.
52. Deer TR, Mekhail N, Provenzano D, Pope J, Krames E, Leong M, et al. The appropriate use of neurostimulation of the spinal cord and peripheral nervous system for the treatment of chronic pain and ischemic diseases: the neuromodulation appropriateness consensus committee. Neuromodulation. 2014;17:515–50.

53. North R, Shipley J, Prager J, Barolat G, Barulich M, Bedder M, et al. Practice parameters for the use of spinal cord stimulation in the treatment of chronic neuropathic pain. Pain Med [Internet]. 2007 [cited 2015 May 17];8 Suppl 4:S200–75. Available from: http://www.ncbi.nlm.nih.gov/pubmed/17995571.
54. Williams KA, Gonzalez-Fernandez M, Hamzehzadeh S, Wilkinson I, Erdek MA, Plunkett A, et al. A multi-center analysis evaluating factors associated with spinal cord stimulation outcome in chronic pain patients. Pain Med. 2011;12:1142–53.
55. Bennett G, Burchiel K, Buchser E, Classen A, Deer T, Du Pen S, et al. Clinical guidelines for intraspinal infusion: report of an expert panel. PolyAnalgesic Consensus Conference 2000. J Pain Symptom Manage [Internet]. 2000 [cited 2015 May 23];20:S37–43. Available from: http://www.ncbi.nlm.nih.gov/pubmed/10989256.
56. Boswell MV, Trescot AM, Datta S, Schultz DM, Hansen HC, Abdi S, et al. Interventional techniques: evidence-based practice guidelines in the management of chronic spinal pain. Pain Physician. 2007;10:7–111.

Chapter 6
Considerations for Neuromodulation

Jeffrey S. Berger

Key Points

- Despite rapidly evolving technology and significantly increased utilization, the complication rate associated with neuromodulation therapies, as well as explant rates remain an issue.
- There are multiple medical factors including anticoagulation status, diabetes and immunocompromised states, bacterial colonization, prior surgical incisions, tobacco use, obesity, and potential for pregnancy which should be considered prior to pursuing neuromodulation therapy.
- Device-related factors including MRI compatibility, componentry allergy as well as pacemaker status need to be properly considered and addressed to ensure successful future outcome and reduce risk of explant.
- SCS and intrathecal catheter/pump implants involve the neuroaxis and as such more conservative anticoagulation discontinuation guidelines have been developed for these procedures in comparison to injectional procedures.
- Tight postoperative glycemic control, screening for and treating *S. aureus* colonization as well as tobacco cessation have all been demonstrated to reduce complication rates.
- MRI compatible componentry is now available from all of the major device manufacturers. While all SCS manufacturers continue to maintain warnings regarding possible interactions, the presence of a pacemaker/ICD is generally a consideration rather than a strict contraindication to SCS therapy.

J.S. Berger, D.O. (✉)
Sports and Spine Rehabilitation Division, Premier Orthopaedic & Sports Medicine,
1204 Baltimore Pike, Suite 100, Chadds Ford, PA 19317, USA
e-mail: jberger@premierortho.com

© Springer International Publishing Switzerland 2016
S.M. Falowski, J.E. Pope (eds.), *Integrating Pain Treatment into Your Spine Practice*, DOI 10.1007/978-3-319-27796-7_6

Introduction

Over the course of 50 years, there have been remarkable advances in the field of neuromodulation. Since the first report by Shealy, Mortimer, and Reswick on the use of pacemaker technology to stimulate the spinal cord to ameliorate cancer-related pain, there have been tremendous advances in electrode, lead as well as implantable pulse generator (IPG) technology [1]. With improved componentry, physicians are equipped with treatment options for a growing range of pain syndromes ranging from failed back surgery syndrome to complex regional pain syndrome (CRPS) to peripheral vascular disease as well as visceral pain states. Improved trialing and implantation technique as well componentry has led to a significant reduction in biologic complications as well as device-related malfunction [2–4].

Enhanced technology, reduced complication rate, improved physician education, and growing community awareness have opened the door to treatment for tens of thousands of patients who previously had no options outside of "living with the pain." Spinal cord stimulation (SCS) is increasingly being recognized as an under-utilized treatment of chronic pain syndromes such as failed back surgery syndrome (FBSS) yet often remains relegated as a treatment of last resort [5, 6]. Factors such as pregnancy, ICD (pacemaker/defibrillator) status, or need for future MRIs which previously have been identified as contraindications now are deemed considerations [7–13]. Traditionally, neurostimulation has been indicated for neuropathic pain states involving the lower limbs; increasingly SCS and PNS are being successfully utilized for treatment of axial low back pain, cancer-related pain, peripheral vascular disease as well as less traditional applications such as knee pain, angina, chronic abdominal as well as pelvic pain [14–18].

With improved technology, increased awareness, and earlier implementation in the treatment algorithm, the utilization of neuromodulation has significantly increased over the past 20 years with exponential growth in the number of trials as well as permanent implants. However, a recent national study of 21,672 patients undergoing spinal cord stimulator trials between 2000 and 2009 identified a trial to permanent conversion ratio of only 41.4 % [7].

As the pool of potential neuromodulation candidates increases, it is critical that neuromodulators take into consideration modifiable and nonmodifiable medical and psychological factors as well as device-related considerations which ultimately will predict trial success, long-term patient satisfaction, as well as risk of complication and associated morbidity. This chapter focuses on biologic and device-related considerations for selecting appropriate candidates for neuromodulation, optimizing outcomes, and reducing modifiable risk factors.

Biologic Considerations

The complication rate associated with spinal cord stimulation has been reported to range between 30 and 40 % [2, 4]. Complications associated with neuromodulation may be mechanical in nature related to lead fracture, lead migration or implantable pulse generator (IPG) failure, biologic related to infection, allergic reaction, IPG seroma, epidural fibrosis, epidural hematoma or physiologic related to change in stimulation coverage, dural puncture, nerve or cord injury, or compressive pathology [2].

Identifying appropriate candidates for neuromodulation is the key to successful outcomes. Once it has been determined that the topography and morphology of a patient's pain state may respond to neurostimulation, neuromodulators must take a thorough history and perform a complete physical examination to determine medical comorbidities that may influence componentry selection as well as risks associated with the trial and permanent implant. Medical considerations reviewed in this chapter include anticoagulation, diabetes and immunocompromised states, bacterial colonization, prior surgical incisions, tobacco use, obesity, pregnancy as well as need for future MRIs.

Anticoagulation

One of the most devastating complications of neuromodulation is development of epidural hematoma, subsequent cord compression, myelopathy, and paralysis. The risk of bleeding-related complications associated with neuraxial anesthesia is significantly greater in patients on anticoagulation therapy and clear, evidence-based guidelines have been developed [19]. The majority of guidelines in this area have been adopted from the anesthesia literature and until recently few evidence-based guidelines existed for physicians performing interventional spine therapies including spinal cord stimulation [20]. In contrast, the role of antithrombotic therapy in preventing cardiovascular and cardio-embolic events has been well established and well researched with multiple large evidence-based trials and secondary guidelines for use and discontinuation [21–23]. The risks of myocardial infarction, pulmonary embolism, stroke, and death associated with holding anticoagulation must be balanced with the increased risk of epidural, pocket, or incisional hematoma and operative blood loss. Some patients such as those with recent cardiac stenting, active cardiac arrhythmia, or thromboembolic event may be deemed too high risk to discontinue therapy. In addition, increased psychological stress associated with the chronic pain syndrome may further increase the rate of thromboembolism by contributing to a state of relative hypercoagulability [24].

Consideration should be given toward reducing the duration of spinal cord stimulator trials to 5 days or less in patients at risk for thromboembolic event who are holding anticoagulation therapy [25]. Due to decision-making complexity associated with ever-growing numbers of drugs, drug classes, and disease states, well-coordinated communication with the patient's hematologist, cardiologist, or prescribing physician is essential to determine whether the patient is at an acceptable risk to hold therapy and mitigate risks associated with doing so. Whenever possible, written authorization including documentation of specific medications, hold duration, and need for bridging therapy is advised.

The risk of spinal hematoma, defined as symptomatic bleeding within the neuraxial space, has been estimated to be less than 1:150,000 based on 13 identified cases of spinal hematoma associated with 850,000 injections of epidural anesthetics [19, 26]. When performed on patients on low molecular weight heparin (LMWH), the risk of spinal hematoma has been estimated to be unacceptably high at greater than 1:3000 [19, 27]. The risk of bleeding is greatest during initial placement and subsequent removal of the neurostimulation leads. Difficult lead access, placement of multiple leads, multiple attempts at epidural access, difficulty guiding the lead to target location as well as physician inexperience may all increase the risk of spinal hematoma. The use of large gauge needles with long bevels, decreased lead pliability related to stiff inner stylettes as well as longer duration trials may further escalate these risk rates.

The American Society for Regional Anesthesia (ASRA) guidelines for discontinuing antithrombotic and thrombolytic therapy have traditionally been used as a surrogate in guiding decision-making. A recent study however indicated that 98 % of respondents followed ASRA guidelines for anticoagulants but 67 % followed alternate protocols for antiplatelet medications with 55 % discontinuing aspirin (ASA) prior to SCS trials despite recommendations to the contrary [28]. The 2015 ASRA guidelines for interventional spine and pain procedures consider both SCS and intrathecal catheter/pump implants to be high-risk neuraxial procedures and as such advise more conservative discontinuation guidelines for these procedures. For spinal cord stimulator trials patients should hold anticoagulation for appropriate duration both prior to and during the length of the trial [2].

Discontinuation recommendations for neuromodulation procedures now exist for ASA and ASA combinations when used for primary prophylaxis along with phosphodiesterase inhibitors, new anticoagulants (dabigatran, apixaban, rivaroxaban) as well as non-aspirin NSAIDs (excluding celecoxib). For ASA and ASA combinations being employed for secondary prevention, a shared assessment and risk stratification is recommended prior to discontinuing. Patients on warfarin should hold therapy for at least 5 days prior to procedure and a normal preoperative INR is advised (previous general guidelines recommended INR <1.5). Refer to Table 6.1 for a summary of specific recommendations adapted from the 2015 ASRA guidelines for Interventional Spine and Pain Procedures [28].

Diabetes Mellitus

It is well known that patients suffering from diabetes have higher levels of operative risks and surgical complications. Patients with diabetes are considered to be in an immunocompromised state with significantly higher incidence of infection including cystitis, cellulitis, and postoperative wound infection when compared to matched controls [29, 30]. The increased risk of complication associated with diabetes is related to both glycemic influence on immune function along with the long-term effects of hyperglycemia on microvasculature and collagen formation with a subsequent tendency toward impaired wound healing [30].

While no studies specific to neuromodulation have been performed examining complication rates associated with hyperglycemia, multiple studies have demonstrated that diabetes is an independent factor predicting postoperative infection risk.

Table 6.1 Recommendations regarding discontinuation of anticoagulation therapy for neuromodulation patients based on 2015 ASRA Guidelines for Interventional Spine and Pain Procedures

Medication	Recommendation
Non-aspirin NSAIDs (excluding celecoxib)	Discontinue 5 half-lives prior to procedure. Restart 2 h after procedure
ASA, ASA combinations for primary prophylaxis	Discontinue 6 days prior to procedure. Restart 24 h after procedure
Phosphodiesterase inhibitors (Cilostazol, Dipyridamole)	Discontinue 2 days prior to procedure. Restart 24 h after procedure
Anticoagulants	
Warfarin	Discontinue 5 days prior to procedure, normal pre-op INR. Restart 24 h after procedure
Acenocoumarol	Discontinue 3 days prior to procedure, normal pre-op INR. Restart 24 h after procedure
IV Heparin	Discontinue 4 h prior to procedure. Restart 2 h after procedure
SQ Heparin, BID and TID	Discontinue 8–10 h prior to procedure. Restart 2 h after procedure
LMWH (prophylactic)	Discontinue 12 h prior to procedure. Restart 12–24 h after procedure
LMWH (therapeutic)	Discontinue 24 h prior to procedure. Restart 12–24 h after procedure
Fibrinolytics: Fondaparinux	Discontinue 4 days prior to procedure. Restart 24 h after procedure
New anticoagulants	
Dabigatran	Discontinue 4–5 days prior to procedure (6 days in patients with impaired renal function). Restart 24 h after procedure
Apixaban	Discontinue 3–5 days prior to procedure. Restart 12–24 h after procedure
Rivaroxaban	Discontinue 3 days prior to procedure. Restart 24 h after procedure
P2Y12 inhibitors	
Clopidogrel	Discontinue 7 days prior to procedure. Restart 12–24 h after procedure
Prasugrel	Discontinue 7–10 days prior to procedure. Restart 12–24 h after procedure
Ticagrelor	Discontinue 5 days prior to procedure. Restart 12–24 h after procedure
Glycoprotein IIb/IIIa inhibitors	
Abciximab	Discontinue 2–5 days prior to procedure. Restart 8–12 h after procedure
Eptifibatide	Discontinue 8–24 h prior to procedure. Restart 8–12 h after procedure
Tirofiban	Discontinue 8–24 h prior to procedure. Restart 8–12 h after procedure
Antidepressants and serotonin reuptake inhibitors (SRIs)	Discontinuation for a period of 1–2 weeks; only necessary in high-risk patients with stable depression (5 weeks for fluoxetine)

Data from Narouze S, et al. Interventional spine and pain procedures in patients on antiplatelet and anticoagulant medications: guidelines from the American Society of Regional Anesthesia and Pain Medicine, the European Society of Regional Anaesthesia and Pain Therapy, the American Academy of Pain Medicine, the International Neuromodulation Society, the North American Neuromodulation Society, and the World Institute of Pain. Reg Anesth Pain Med. 2015;40(3):182–212

After controlling for all other factors, Golden et al. found that patients with mean blood glucose values >200 mg/dl within 36 h of surgery were at significantly greater risk of postoperative infection. Compared to the lowest quartile blood sugars, patients in each subsequent blood sugar quartile demonstrated increasing rates of infection [30]. Tight glycemic control during the immediate preoperative and ensuing 36 h postoperative period was highly recommended as a modifiable risk factor to reduce the rate of infection and wound-related complications. As the rate of diabetes increases, more patients are expected to seek out neuromodulation for treatment of diabetes-related morbidities such as peripheral polyneuropathy and peripheral vascular disease. When considering neurostimulation, the presence of controlled diabetes represents a consideration rather than a contraindication for neuromodulation therapies, and patients should be educated regarding risks of postoperative hyperglycemia with implementation of aggressive glycemic control interventions.

Tobacco Use

Active smoking has been identified as an independent risk factor contributing to the development of low back pain, and the incidence of tobacco use is generally greater in the patients with chronic pain [31]. Therefore, there is likely a higher incidence of smoking in patients being considered for neuromodulation therapy. Multiple randomized controlled and prospective cohort studies have demonstrated that smoking results in impaired wound healing in "clean" skin wounds. These same studies have identified that a short period of smoking abstinence reduces the risk of wound infection back to the levels of nonsmoker controls. The use of nicotine replacement therapies such as a nicotine patch has not been demonstrated to increase the rate of surgical site infection (SSI) [32]. Smoking cessation for a period of at least 3 weeks prior to surgery has been found to significantly reduce the risk of postoperative impaired wound healing as well as infection for head and neck surgery. In a randomized controlled study evaluating the effect of smoking cessation on complications related to hip and knee surgery, Moller identified significant reductions in wound-related complications, cardiovascular complications, and secondary surgery with preoperative smoking cessation for a period of 6–8 weeks with an overall complication rate of 18 % in the smoking cessation intervention group versus 52 % in the control group [33]. The beneficial effects of smoking cessation are only maintained with complete abstinence from smoking. While no studies exist specifically evaluating the effect of tobacco use on neuromodulation therapies, similar deleterious effects on neuromodulation implants can be extrapolated based on a number of studies evaluating a diversity of operative interventions [32–34]. While active tobacco use is not an absolute contraindication to neuromodulation therapy, it represents an independent risk factor for wound-related complications. As such, potential neuromodulation candidates should be educated regarding the deleterious effects of smoking on wound healing, and counseled accordingly based on the presence of concomitant risk factors such as diabetes, immunocompromise as well as obesity. All patients should be strongly encouraged to quit smoking altogether or at a minimum abstain from tobacco for a minimum of 3 weeks prior to surgery.

Malnutrition and Obesity

A number of studies have demonstrated a link between obesity and a proinflammatory state [35]. Obesity has been reported to be a risk factor for neurostimulation-related complications including SSI [2]. Obesity has not been shown to be an independent risk factor for accidental dural puncture during epidural anesthesia [36]. Obesity has been linked to a greater complication rate in adults undergoing spinal deformity correction surgery with a higher incidence of major complication as well as SSI [37]. Given the nature of neuromodulation procedures, access to the epidural space may be more difficult in obese individuals with longer operative times which in turn may be linked to greater risk of complication and infection. As such, obese patients should be counseled regarding the potentially elevated risk of major complication as well as infection. Whenever possible weight loss should be encouraged to reduce not only surgical risks but also the multitude of other risks associated with obesity. In obese individuals a goal for successful outcome following neuromodulation should be an increase in activity levels, which may lead to secondary weight loss. Therefore, while not a contraindication, obesity represents another consideration which should be weighed in accordance with other risk factors.

Morbid obesity and malnutrition are often two co-occurring, potentially modifiable risk factors for surgical intervention. Poor nutritional status has been associated with greater risk of serious adverse event following orthopedic surgery [38, 39]. Modifying preoperative risks related to morbid obesity may take longer and prove more difficult than those associated with preoperative malnutrition. Malnutrition as measured by low albumin levels (<3.5 g/dl) has been demonstrated to be associated with greater risk of major perioperative complication when compared to morbid obesity in a large cohort study of patients undergoing total knee arthroplasty. Malnutrition has been associated with increased risk of major complication including mortality, superficial and deep infection, prolonged ventilator time, pneumonia, and renal insufficiency/failure [39]. Preoperative assessment for hypoalbuminemia with appropriate supplementation may be a reasonable consideration for neuromodulation candidates who are at greater risk for malnutrition, particularly if other surgical risk factors are present.

Bacterial Colonization

Staphylococcus aureus is the most common pathogen associated with SSI and is responsible for approximately 25 % of nosocomial infections in the USA. Community studies indicate that 25–30 % of the population at any point in time may be colonized with *S. aureus* in the anterior nares [40–42]. Patients colonized with *S. aureus* may have a two- to tenfold greater risk of developing an SSI [43]. The overall infection risk associated with SCS implantation has been reported to range from 3.4 to 4.6 % which is significant considering the elective nature of the therapy, particularly when compared to lower incidence identified in the pacemaker literature [2, 4, 44].

In a large randomized, controlled study, preoperative screening for *S. aureus* and subsequent intranasal application of mupirocin ointment to colonized individuals did not reduce the risk of SSI, but was shown to significantly reduce the incidence of nosocomial infection [40]. As such, assessment for *S. aureus* colonization and subsequent treatment with mupirocin nasal ointment and chlorhexidine soap may reduce overall infection risk and should be a consideration prior to operative intervention.

Prior Incision Sites

Failed back surgery syndrome is a leading indication in the USA for neuromodulation therapies. When large midline incisions are employed for prior lumbar surgeries or during SCS/PNS lead or IPG revision surgery, it may be necessary to operate at the site of a prior incision. In a large retrospective analysis of predictive factors for complications following general surgery, operating through a prior incision was identified in 32 % of patients with postoperative wound infection [45]. Operating at the site of a previous incision may predispose to infection as a result of decreased vascularity in scar tissue. Operating through a previous incision may also be associated with more complicated procedures necessitating longer surgical times which in turn is also associated with greater infection risk [45]. When possible, neuromodulators should avoid operating through prior incision sites and should give consideration to utilizing alternate IPG sites for revision surgery, particularly in patients with a history of infection or multiple risk factors.

Pregnancy

As the number of patients undergoing neurostimulation therapy for chronic pain increases, a growing number of case studies have been reported in the literature examining the use of SCS during pregnancy. Women of child-bearing age may have the highest incidence of complex regional pain syndrome (CRPS) [46] for which SCS has been demonstrated as an effective form of treatment [47]. Many of these women rely on SCS to maintain functional lives and reduce or avoid the burden of opioid or anticonvulsant medications which may pose risk to the developing fetus [48]. As a result of chronic pain and medication reliance, many women are not even able to consider the possibility of pregnancy until after successful treatment with neurostimulation therapies.

Outside of several case reports, there are no large, controlled studies evaluating maternal and fetal safety in conjunction with the use of a previously implanted SCS device during pregnancy [7, 9, 48]. While no case report to date has identified a fetal, maternal, or congenital defect or complication directly attributable to SCS during pregnancy or labor, the small sample size and observational nature of these reports provide little concrete data upon which to base recommendations. When considering neuromodulation therapy for women of child-bearing age, implications for future pregnancy should be discussed and patients should be counseled regarding the lack of concrete, longitudinal data.

Device-Related Considerations

MRI Compatibility

In the past many patient who would otherwise be excellent candidates for neuro-stimulation were excluded based on potential need for magnetic resonance imaging (MRI) to monitor disease states. Starting in 2013, manufacturers have received FDA approval for MRI compatibility. Medtronic offers full-body 1.5 T MRI compatibility with spinal cord stimulation systems using both percutaneous and surgical paddle leads. St. Jude, Boston Scientific, and Nevro have MRI compatible componentry enabling MRI of the brain and extremities. Still, limitations exist with regard to MRI safety in patients with SCS, including those patients needing access to high magnetic field MRI. In patients with diseases such as multiple sclerosis with need for routine MRI monitoring, communication with the patient's neurologist should take place when considering candidacy for SCS/PNS.

Allergy

Multiple cases of allergic reaction to pacemakers and associated componentry have been reported in the literature [49]. Several case reports documenting allergic reaction, contact sensitivity to SCS has been reported [50, 51]. Symptoms related to allergic reaction may include itching, swelling, rash, or malaise [50] and may respond to corticosteroids. Given similar presentation to infection, this is a likely under-recognized complication frequently misdiagnosed as infection. In patients with known allergy to titanium, platinum, iridium, or polyurethane or a history of multiple contact sensitivities, skin patch testing can be obtained from the manufacturer [2].

Pacemaker Status

In the past, the use of SCS/PNS in conjunction with pacemakers or implantable cardioverter defibrillator (ICD) represented a clear contraindication. This was related to concern regarding possible false inhibition of pacemaker or false activation of ICD as a result of SCS impulses [12]. Subsequently, multiple case reports emerged in the literature demonstrating safety with combined usage of these two devices [11–13]. While all SCS manufacturers continue to maintain warnings regarding possible interactions between these devices, the presence of a pacemaker/ICD is generally considered to be a consideration rather than a strict contraindication to SCS therapy. In patients with pacemakers and/or ICD, communication and coordination should take place with the patient's cardiologist and a pacemaker device representative should be available to assess for inappropriate feedback between devices. Prior to pursuing neurostimulation, pacemaker/ICD patients should be counseled that despite the fact that no cases of adverse interaction between devices have been reported, theoretical concerns regarding feedback between devices may still exist.

Summary

Enhanced technology, reduced complication rate, improved physician education, and growing community awareness have led to a dramatic rise in the number of patients being treated with neuromodulation therapies. When selecting appropriate candidates for neuromodulation, there are a number of biologic and device related factors that physicians should evaluate and address when possible prior to operative intervention. These can include potential risk factors for perioperative and postoperative complications such as anticoagulation and antiplatelet therapy, diabetes mellitus, tobacco use, bacterial colonization, prior incision sites, obesity, as well as malnutrition. Device related factors including MRI compatibility, use in conjunction with pacemakers/ICDS, as well as implications for future pregnancy need to be appropriately stratified and counseled. When these factors are properly identified, patients can be appropriately counseled and modifiable risk factors addressed to ensure best possible outcomes with neuromodulation therapy.

References

1. Shealy CN, Mortimer JT, Reswick JB. Electrical inhibition of pain by stimulation of the dorsal columns: preliminary clinical report. Anesth Analg. 1967;46(4):489–91.
2. Deer TR, Mekhail N, Provenzano D, Pope J, Krames E, Thomson S, et al. The appropriate use of neurostimulation: avoidance and treatment of complications of neurostimulation therapies for the treatment of chronic pain. Neuromodulation Appropriateness Consensus Committee. Neuromodulation. 2014;17(6):571–97. discussion 597–8.
3. Kumar K, Buchser E, Linderoth B, Meglio M, Van Buyten J-P. Avoiding complications from spinal cord stimulation: practical recommendations from an international panel of experts. Neuromodulation. 2007;10(1):24–33.
4. Cameron T. Safety and efficacy of spinal cord stimulation for the treatment of chronic pain: a 20-year literature review. J Neurosurg. 2004;100(3 Suppl Spine):254–67.
5. Lad SP, Babu R, Bagley JH, Choi J, Bagley CA, Huh BK, et al. Utilization of spinal cord stimulation in patients with failed back surgery syndrome. Spine. 2014;39(12):E719–27.
6. Krames ES, Monis S, Poree L, Deer T, Levy R. Using the SAFE principles when evaluating electrical stimulation therapies for the pain of failed back surgery syndrome. Neuromodulation. 2011;14(4):299–311.
7. Bernardini DJ, Pratt SD, Takoudes TC, Simopoulos TT. Spinal cord stimulation and the pregnant patient-specific considerations for management: a case series and review of the literature. Neuromodulation. 2010;13(4):270–4.
8. Saxena A, Eljamel MS. Spinal cord stimulation in the first two trimesters of pregnancy: case report and review of the literature. Neuromodulation. 2009;12(4):281–3.
9. Segal R. Spinal cord stimulation, conception, pregnancy, and labor: case study in a complex regional pain syndrome patient. Neuromodulation. 1999;2(1):41–5.

10. Ekre O, Borjesson M, Edvardsson N, Eliasson T, Mannheimer C. Feasibility of spinal cord stimulation in angina pectoris in patients with chronic pacemaker treatment for cardiac arrhythmias. Pacing Clin Electrophysiol. 2003;26(11):2134–41.
11. Ooi YC, Falowski S, Wang D, Jallo J, Ho RT, Sharan A. Simultaneous use of neurostimulators in patients with a preexisting cardiovascular implantable electronic device. Neuromodulation. 2011;14(1):20–5. discussion 25–6.
12. Kosharskyy B, Rozen D. Feasibility of spinal cord stimulation in a patient with a cardiac pacemaker. Pain Physician. 2006;9(3):249–51.
13. Romano M, Brusa S, Grieco A, Zucco F, Spinelli A, Allaria B. Efficacy and safety of permanent cardiac DDD pacing with contemporaneous double spinal cord stimulation. Pacing Clin Electrophysiol. 1998;21(2):465–7.
14. Falco FJE, Berger J, Vrable A, Onyewu O, Zhu J. Cross talk: a new method for peripheral nerve stimulation. An observational report with cadaveric verification. Pain Physician. 2009;12(6):965–83.
15. Lihua P, Su M, Zejun Z, Ke W, Bennett MI. Spinal cord stimulation for cancer-related pain in adults. Cochrane Database Syst Rev. 2013;2.
16. Deogaonkar M, Zibly Z, Slavin KV. Spinal cord stimulation for the treatment of vascular pathology. Neurosurg Clin N Am. 2014;25(1):25–31.
17. Hunter C, Dave N, Diwan S, Deer T. Neuromodulation of pelvic visceral pain: review of the literature and case series of potential novel targets for treatment. Pain Pract. 2013;13(1):3–17.
18. McRoberts WP, Roche M. Novel approach for peripheral subcutaneous field stimulation for the treatment of severe, chronic knee joint pain after total knee arthroplasty. Neuromodulation. 2010;13(2):131–6.
19. Horlocker TT, Wedel DJ, Rowlingson JC, Enneking FK, Kopp SL, Benzon HT, et al. Regional anesthesia in the patient receiving antithrombotic or thrombolytic therapy: American Society of Regional Anesthesia and Pain Medicine Evidence-Based Guidelines (Third Edition). Reg Anesth Pain Med. 2010;35(1):64–101.
20. Manchikanti L, Abdi S, Atluri S, Benyamin RM, Boswell MV, Buenaventura RM, et al. An update of comprehensive evidence-based guidelines for interventional techniques in chronic spinal pain. Part II: guidance and recommendations. Pain Physician. 2013;16(2 Suppl):S49–283.
21. Biondi-Zoccai GGL, Lotrionte M, Agostoni P, Abbate A, Fusaro M, Burzotta F, et al. A systematic review and meta-analysis on the hazards of discontinuing or not adhering to aspirin among 50,279 patients at risk for coronary artery disease. Eur Heart J. 2006;27(22):2667–74.
22. Thachil J, Gatt A, Martlew V. Management of surgical patients receiving anticoagulation and antiplatelet agents. Br J Surg. 2008;95(12):1437–48.
23. Geerts WH, Bergqvist D, Pineo GF, Heit JA, Samama CM, Lassen MR, et al. Prevention of venous thromboembolism: American College of Chest Physicians Evidence-Based Clinical Practice Guidelines (8th Edition). Chest. 2008;133(6 Suppl):381S–453.
24. von Kanel R, Mills PJ, Fainman C, Dimsdale JE. Effects of psychological stress and psychiatric disorders on blood coagulation and fibrinolysis: a biobehavioral pathway to coronary artery disease? Psychosom Med. 2001;63(4):531–44.
25. Chincholkar M, Eldabe S, Strachan R, Brookes M, Garner F, Chadwick R, et al. Prospective analysis of the trial period for spinal cord stimulation treatment for chronic pain. Neuromodulation. 2011;14(6):523–8. discussion 528–9.
26. Tryba M. [Epidural regional anesthesia and low molecular heparin: Pro]. Anasthesiol Intensivmed Notfallmed Schmerzther. 1993;28(3):179–81.
27. Schroeder DR. Statistics: detecting a rare adverse drug reaction using spontaneous reports. Reg Anesth Pain Med. 1998;23(6 Suppl 2):183–9.
28. Narouze S, Benzon HT, Provenzano DA, Buvanendran A, De Andres J, Deer TR, et al. Interventional spine and pain procedures in patients on antiplatelet and anticoagulant medications: guidelines from the American Society of Regional Anesthesia and Pain Medicine, the European Society of Regional Anaesthesia and Pain Therapy, the American Academy of Pain Medicine, the International Neuromodulation Society, the North American Neuromodulation Society, and the World Institute of Pain. Reg Anesth Pain Med. 2015;40(3):182–212.

29. Chen SL, Jackson SL, Boyko EJ. Diabetes mellitus and urinary tract infection: epidemiology, pathogenesis and proposed studies in animal models. J Urol. 2009;182(6 Suppl):S51–6.
30. Golden SH, Peart-Vigilance C, Kao WH, Brancati FL. Perioperative glycemic control and the risk of infectious complications in a cohort of adults with diabetes. Diabetes Care. 1999;22(9):1408–14.
31. Claus M, Kimbel R, Spahn D, Dudenhoffer S, Rose D-M, Letzel S. Prevalence and influencing factors of chronic back pain among staff at special schools with multiple and severely handicapped children in Germany: results of a cross-sectional study. BMC Musculoskelet Disord. 2014;15:55.
32. Yang GP, Longaker MT. Abstinence from smoking reduces incisional wound infection: a randomized, controlled trial. Ann Surg. 2003;238(1):1–5.
33. Moller AM, Villebro N, Pedersen T, Tonnesen H. Effect of preoperative smoking intervention on postoperative complications: a randomised clinical trial. Lancet. 2002;359(9301):114–7.
34. Kuri M, Nakagawa M, Tanaka H, Hasuo S, Kishi Y. Determination of the duration of preoperative smoking cessation to improve wound healing after head and neck surgery. Anesthesiology. 2005;102(5):892–6.
35. Pence BD, Woods JA. Exercise, obesity, and cutaneous wound healing: evidence from rodent and human studies. Adv Wound Care. 2014;3(1):71–9.
36. Kuroda K, Miyoshi H, Kato T, Nakamura R, Yasuda T, Oshita K, et al. Factors related to accidental dural puncture in epidural anesthesia patients. J Clin Anesth. 2015;27(8):665–7. http://www.ncbi.nlm.nih.gov/pubmed/26230419.
37. Soroceanu A, Burton DC, Diebo BG, Smith JS, Hostin R, Shaffrey CI, et al. Impact of obesity on complications, infection, and patient-reported outcomes in adult spinal deformity surgery. J Neurosurg Spine. 2015;31:1–9.
38. Jensen JE, Jensen TG, Smith TK, Johnston DA, Dudrick SJ. Nutrition in orthopaedic surgery. J Bone Joint Surg Am. 1982;64(9):1263–72.
39. Nelson CL, Elkassabany NM, Kamath AF, Liu J. Low albumin levels, more than morbid obesity, are associated with complications after TKA. Clin Orthop. 2015;473(10):3163–72.
40. Perl TM, Cullen JJ, Wenzel RP, Zimmerman MB, Pfaller MA, Sheppard D, et al. Intranasal mupirocin to prevent postoperative Staphylococcus aureus infections. N Engl J Med. 2002;346(24):1871–7.
41. Bode LGM, Kluytmans JAJW, Wertheim HFL, Bogaers D, Vandenbroucke-Grauls CMJE, Roosendaal R, et al. Preventing surgical-site infections in nasal carriers of Staphylococcus aureus. N Engl J Med. 2010;362(1):9–17.
42. Kluytmans J, van Belkum A, Verbrugh H. Nasal carriage of Staphylococcus aureus: epidemiology, underlying mechanisms, and associated risks. Clin Microbiol Rev. 1997;10(3):505–20.
43. Perl TM, Golub JE. New approaches to reduce Staphylococcus aureus nosocomial infection rates: treating S. aureus nasal carriage. Ann Pharmacother. 1998;32(1):S7–16.
44. Turner JA, Loeser JD, Deyo RA, Sanders SB. Spinal cord stimulation for patients with failed back surgery syndrome or complex regional pain syndrome: a systematic review of effectiveness and complications. Pain. 2004;108(1–2):137–47.
45. Triantafyllopoulos G, Stundner O, Memtsoudis S, Poultsides LA. Patient, surgery, and hospital related risk factors for surgical site infections following total hip arthroplasty. ScientificWorldJournal. 2015;2015:979560.
46. Schwartzman RJ, Erwin KL, Alexander GM. The natural history of complex regional pain syndrome. Clin J Pain. 2009;25(4):273–80.
47. Sanders RA, Moeschler SM, Gazelka HM, Lamer TJ, Wang Z, Qu W, et al. Patient outcomes and spinal cord stimulation: a retrospective case series evaluating patient satisfaction, pain scores, and opioid requirements. Pain Pract. 2015. doi:10.1111/papr.12340.
48. Young AC, Lubenow TR, Buvanendran A. The parturient with implanted spinal cord stimulator: management and review of the literature. Reg Anesth Pain Med. 2015;40(3):276–83.
49. Abdallah HI, Balsara RK, O'Riordan AC. Pacemaker contact sensitivity: clinical recognition and management. Ann Thorac Surg. 1994;57(4):1017–8.
50. Ochani TD, Almirante J, Siddiqui A, Kaplan R. Allergic reaction to spinal cord stimulator. Clin J Pain. 2000;16(2):178–80.
51. Taverner MG. A case of an allergic reaction to a spinal cord stimulator: identification of the antigen with epicutaneous patch testing, allowing successful reimplantation. Neuromodulation. 2013;16(6):595–9.

Part II
Integrating Pain Management into Practice

Chapter 7
Practice Setup

Steven M. Falowski

Key Points

- Having a SCS placed does not mean that spine surgery cannot be performed in the future. It is a treatment modality for their present pain.
- SCS has class I evidence of its superiority when placed against conventional medical management and against repeat spinal surgery.
- Practice setup for the pain physician and treating surgeon can be variable for these interventions.
- Relationships with pain physicians are crucial in spinal surgery. They are usually the first-line treatment for patients with pain with conventional management prior to surgery. They are also the treating physicians for those patients in chronic pain following spinal surgery.
- SCS is not a last resort therapy, with the literature supporting earlier intervention with appropriate patient selection.

Introduction

The neuromodulation community is based on a multidisciplinary approach that is diverse in its delivery. The pedigree of clinicians that offer and employ neuromodulation in their practice vary from neurosurgeons, orthopedic spine surgeons, and anesthesiologists to neurologists and rehabilitation physicians. For the formal nonsurgical residencies, an ACGME (Accreditation Counsel of Graduate Medical Education)-accredited

S.M. Falowski, M.D. (✉)
Neurosurgery, St. Luke's University Health Network,
701 Ostrum St, Suite 302, Bethlehem, PA 18017, USA
e-mail: sfalowski@gmail.com

© Springer International Publishing Switzerland 2016
S.M. Falowski, J.E. Pope (eds.), *Integrating Pain Treatment into Your Spine Practice*, DOI 10.1007/978-3-319-27796-7_7

fellowship is necessary to become Pain Board Certified. The most common disease indications for spinal cord stimulation (SCS) include FBSS, and complex regional pain syndrome (CRPS). The literature supports that SCS can produce at least 50 % pain relief in 50–60 % of the implanted patients and reduce the use of more medications [1]. Interestingly, with the proper follow-up care, these results can be maintained [1, 2]. Very few other invasive modalities can claim this success rate. In addition to SCS there are other therapies including intrathecal drug delivery (IDD), peripheral nerve stimulation (PNS), peripheral nerve field stimulation (PNfS), as well as kyphoplasty and vertebroplasty which can be implemented into this multidisciplinary approach.

For advanced pain care therapies, it is generally accepted that a trial is performed prior to implant. There are several factors that are important in being aware of these therapies and having access to them for your patients.

Referral Network

A proper referral network is an important component to offer your services in the management of pain patients, being mindful of where in the algorithm you would like your practice to be situated. You can quickly develop a niche by being the spine surgeon in your community who offers these neuromodulation therapies or who can help navigate a pathway to obtain them. Many models exist, with the most common for the surgeon described by a pain physician performing the trial and a surgeon performing the permanent implant. However models do exist with the surgeon performing both the trial and the permanent implant. The other option is working with an interventional pain physician who performs both the trial and permanent implant in whom you can build a referral network allowing you to share patients, but most importantly having therapies available to your patients in chronic pain.

Relationships

It goes without saying, but building relationships with doctors in your referral network is important. It allows your practice to grow, and builds your reputation as a surgeon. Relationships with pain physicians are crucial in spinal surgery, as they are usually the first-line treatment for patients with pain with conventional management prior to surgery. They are also the treating physicians for those patients in chronic pain following spinal surgery.

Pain Physicians' and Surgeons' Roles

As a surgeon, your role determines the surgical procedure and the postoperative care, and influences the longitudinal implementation of the therapy. In the realm of interventional pain therapies, such as SCS, there are variable relationships. A common setup includes surgeons who identify patients as either surgical candidates or those who are candidates for SCS. For those patients who are not spinal surgery candidates, a pain physician may then perform a trial of the therapy and either move on to permanent implantation or refer the patient back to the surgeon for permanent implantation. Obviously, communication between the two providers, regarding contact and lead placement that yielded the most efficacious treatment, along with supporting documentation, will help mitigate poor outcomes.

By developing a strong relationship with pain physicians you can determine the roles that work mutually for both sides. A common referral to a spine surgeon in this setting leads to a "surgery versus spinal cord stimulation evaluation." This fosters the most appropriate therapy for the patient. The relationship can span those patients who have undergone spinal surgery and subsequently have ongoing pain following a technically successful surgery or those patients who have not undergone previous surgery. Candidates for SCS or spinal surgery in this setting are most reliably identified from their surgeon.

Patient Identification Is Crucial

As with any spinal procedure, patient selection is paramount in success. Determining proper candidates for pain therapies is crucial.

Early Intervention

It is well known that early intervention in chronic pain is of crucial importance. SCS should not be viewed as a "last resort" therapy. It is important to view it as part of the treatment paradigm. The literature supports that earlier intervention with SCS leads to improved outcomes [3]. As the surgeon you can help drive these therapies in an earlier fashion as you have the most exposure to the patient in the first 6 months following a spinal procedure.

Benefits to Surgeons

As described, it is important to know that literature has shown that 40 % or more of spinal patients will carry the diagnosis of FBSS. This constitutes a large amount of patients within a spine practice that can benefit from these therapies, which have class I evidence to support its use [1, 4]. If you choose the role as an implanting surgeon, not only would offering these therapies substantially increase your case volume and reimbursement, but it will also help you build a niche in your market which will build your referral base, common referrals being evaluation for surgery versus a SCS which helps build your practice on both ends. As an implanting surgeon you may share responsibility with pain physicians in your community who can maintain management of the patient, while you maintain management and responsibility of the SCS implant. Lastly, regardless of the role you choose, it gives you the ability to have options for your patients. This is important as medicine's changing landscape has shifted to patient-centered care.

It is important to realize that your toolbox as a surgeon is based on your knowledge base, technical proficiency, and access to therapies for your patients. By having a working knowledge of these neuromodulation therapies, you will be able to offer the patients what is truly in their best interest, as repeat spinal surgery or even initial spinal surgery is not always the best option [1, 4]. These therapies can be implemented in your practice and increase case volume, maintain the physician–patient relationship, and foster a treatment for the patient over the continuum of their care. Lastly, it is important to realize that these therapies are treatments for their current conditions as spinal surgery may be warranted in the future even after a neuromodulatory intervention.

Summary

Building a neuromodulation and pain practice requires development of expertise and patient access. Providing access to appropriate pain care is essential in the development of a surgeon's practice. Appreciating this paradigm, many patients already in your practice would likely benefit from these neuromodulation modalities. Practice setup can vary, but if integrated into the surgeons' practice would increase case volume and reimbursement, as well as build a niche in your market. Referral networks and relationships in a spine program are crucial for both surgeons and pain physicians alike. Surgeons should be well equipped to perform evaluations for surgery versus an SCS or IDD. In addition surgeons should be knowledgeable of the therapy options available in order to guide their patients, especially in the setting of pain following a spinal surgery. This helps build your practice by developing multiple touch points within a treatment algorithm. As an implanting surgeon, you may share responsibility with pain physicians in your community who can maintain management of the patient, while you maintain management and responsibility of the SCS implant.

References

1. Kumar K, Taylor RS, Jacques L, et al. PROCESS study SCS vs CMM for FBSS pain. Neuromodulation. 2007;132(1–2):179–88.
2. Kumar K, et al. Spinal cord stimulation in treatment of chronic benign pain: challenges in treatment planning and present status, a 22-year experience. Neurosurgery. 2006;58(3):481–96. discussion 481–96.

3. Kumar K, Rizvi S, Nguyen R, Abbas M, Bishop S, Murthy V. Impact of wait times on spinal cord stimulation therapy outcomes. Pain Pract. 2014;14(8):709–20. doi:10.1111/papr.12126. Epub 2013 Oct 25.
4. North RB, Kidd DH, Farrokhi F, Piantadosi SA. SCS vs re-operation for FBSS*. Neurosurgery. 2005;56(1):98–106.

Chapter 8
Referral Networks

Jason E. Pope

Key Points

- The development for a strong referral network improves patient care by expediting delivery of specialty services.
- Careful planning can create an opportunity to assist the patient in navigating the health care system.
- Geographic and resource limitations, both from the patients and the surrounding providers, greatly impact the development model.
- Transparency and communication of expectations are important to convey and revisit.
- Stark and anti-kickback statutes help govern defining some of these interactions.

Introduction

Formal training in medicine suggests that partnerships among specialties to improve the patient's global condition are essential. This concept is inherent to the growth of medicine and its complexity [1], creating the need for specialty management to keep pace. Patients need to have a visible and definable pathway to get efficient and efficacious care, with easily navigable involvement with general practitioners and subspecialties. These relationships among providers define this pathway and serve many functions, both in the clinical and business realms.

J.E. Pope, M.D., D.A.B.P.M., F.I.P.P. (✉)
Summit Pain Alliance, 392 Tesconi Court, Santa Rosa, CA 95401, USA
e-mail: popeje@me.com

© Springer International Publishing Switzerland 2016
S.M. Falowski, J.E. Pope (eds.), *Integrating Pain Treatment into Your Spine Practice*, DOI 10.1007/978-3-319-27796-7_8

Patient Pathway

Referral networks are created based on patient need, access, durability, and outcome of the services rendered.

Provider Referral Model

PATIENT → PROVIDER1 → PROVIDER2 → PROVIDER3

For the case of this example, let's assume that the patient has axial back pain with unilateral lower extremity radicular complaints and no weakness, or numbness, and is 2 months from a lifting injury.

As one might expect, the role of PROVIDER 1 (first to patient) is a complex one, and is based on community resources and services rendered. For example, a patient living in rural West Virginia would likely see their community primary care provider (PCP), where a referral would be made to whomever is the specialty available in the area, which could be a neurologist and physiatrist, pain physician, orthopedic spine surgeon, or a neurosurgeon. The approach and the services offered to the patient are markedly different based on the specialty of the provider. For instance, if the patient were to go to a neurologist, likely physical therapy and neuropathic pain medications would be initiated. Being evaluated by a surgeon would likely lead to a surgical opinion being rendered. If the patient went to a pain physician, likely physical therapy and an epidural would be offered. Depending on the success or failure of the conservative (and geographically regional) care, the patient may need to see another provider to complete the treatment algorithm (PROVIDER 3).

Further, the patient in this rural center is unlikely to seek subspecialty resources for an opinion (PROVIDER 2) first and ultimately bypassing the community primary care provider in this rural setting. If this same patient lived in San Francisco, the reliance on a referral from the PCP is less, creating a potential need for direct-to-patient (or consumer) marketing.

This point of this divergent algorithmic approach can be underscored at a major tertiary care academic facility. One would expect that if a patient called the academic facility with the presentation of the above complaints, they would be routed uniformly through a treatment approach, under the umbrella of care. Indeed, this is not the case, and depending on the operator that answered the phone, the patient could be directed to physiatry, neurosurgery, orthopedic surgery, vascular surgery, pain management, or physical therapy.

The dependence of the patient on this gateway of care is vital to appreciate. Patients will follow the algorithm and treatment pathway their physicians put into motion, demonstrating the importance of having a keen understanding of your position in this algorithm and where to place the patient within the scope of your practice and those in your referral network.

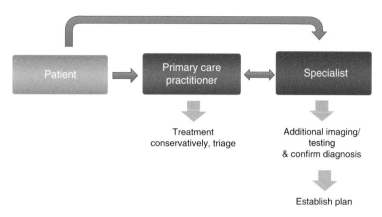

Fig. 8.1 Patient-centric model

As can be expected, the physician's practice setting influences these defined pathways; however, the principles of relationship and network building are the same. The longitudinal philosophy of a linear referral care model is antiquated. The Provider Referral Model has evolved appropriately to look more like Fig. 8.1. Of most change in this evolution is the ability of the patient to have an interchangeable flow between the PCP and specialist that is fluid and easily adjusted.

Referral Networks

When developing a referral network, as illustrated in the example above, a regional analysis of gaps in patient care and opportunity is paramount. This includes patient population demographics (median age, number, major employers, insurance type), services available (number and type of medical entities in the area), specialties that may be in your referral network, and specifically types of practices similar to your own. Marketing firms typically provide this service [2]. Once the architecture of the target is surveyed, work can begin on creating patient access to your clinic.

Essential Networks for Surgeons Providing Pain Care

The surgeon's goal is to operate to improve patient care, with the expectation that patients are appropriately referred and the pathology vetted. Good outcomes are desired, whether the focus is for improved pain or function. Pain care requires a reciprocal relationship with several specialties:

1. Pain Management

    (a) Should be ACGME boarded.
    (b) Background specialties typically include anesthesiology and physiatry/ physical medicine and rehabilitation.

2. Neurology
3. Primary Care
4. Psychiatry and Psychology

Chronic pain, as defined by the International Association for the Study of Pain, is pain that is unresolving after 6 months [3]. With the redistribution of patients away from long-term opioid use, chronic opioid mitigating strategies are paramount to be employed earlier. When simple strategies fail, and patients have nonoperative pathology, advanced pain care therapies can be employed, such as spinal cord stimulation (SCS) [4, 5]. As previously defined in the text, although the candidacy of the patient for neuromodulation can be assessed and determined by many specialties, the trial is typically performed by the pain management physician, and the permanent is performed by a surgeon skilled to perform the permanent procedure.

Defining the Ideal Partnership

Ideal partnerships involve some fairly simple principles, but for the sake of completeness are worth mentioning. These principles include:

1. Respect
2. Transparency
3. Goodwill
4. Patient-focused care
5. Availability for service
6. Communication

The typical worry when referral networks are created is the conception of "losing your patient." In the authors' estimation, this concept is misguided and antiquated. The focus of diligent and vigilant patient care should govern referral patterns. In our previous patient, if the patient is referred to PROVIDER 1, for the sake of our example, a surgeon, after assessment of surgical candidacy, goes to PROVIDER 2, a pain physician, for a trial of conservative care. If conservative therapy fails, and if the doctor-physician relationship is healthy, the patient should return to PROVIDER 1 for reassessment of surgical options. Notwithstanding, the aforementioned is contingent on the requirement that the providers have the expertise and skill to exercise these roles. If the patient is deemed a nonsurgical candidate and SCS is appropriate, then the patient could return to PROVIDER 2 for a trial of therapy. This allows for patient continuity and improvement in outcomes. This concept of a relationship with integration of specialties is paramount in the success of proper patient care, and especially in neuromodulation. This highlights the importance of an open referral network between surgeons and pain physicians and demonstrates that the roles are fluid. Although the surgeon may not find a surgical pathology, they can be involved with the permanent implantation of a spinal cord stimulator, while the pain physician who has performed conservative measures can now exclude a surgical pathology before proceeding with a spinal cord stimulator trial.

Stark and Anti-kickback

No discussion of referral networks is completed without a comment on the laws surrounding physician referrals. Stark law ((42 USC §1395nn)) and anti-kickback laws are designed to keep the focus on the diligent care of the patient [6–8]. A complete review of this topic is beyond the scope of this chapter, and for a detailed discussion it is advised to consult your personal attorney. Essentially, Stark law governs the interaction of referrals from one entity to another owned or operated by a physician (Fig. 8.2).

The federal anti-kickback statute ((42 USC §1320a-7b(b)) is a policy that prohibits the enticement as a reward for referral of federal health care business. For instance, in the example of the patient above, if PROVIDER 1 refers to PROVIDER 2 and receives payment for the referral, this obviously violates anti-kickback statute. Table 8.1 describes the difference.

Fig. 8.2 Stark law

Subpart A—General Exclusions and Exclusion of Particular Services

§411.1 Basis and scope.

(a) *Statutory basis.* Sections 1814(a) and 1835(a) of the Act require that a physician certify or recertify a patient's need for home health services but, in general, prohibit a physician from certifying or recertifying the need for services if the services will be furnished by an HHA in which the physician has a significant ownership interest, or with which the physician has a significant financial or contractual relationship. Sections 1814(c), 1835(d), and 1862 of the Act exclude from Medicare payment certain specified services. The Act provides special rules for payment of services furnished by the following: Federal providers or agencies (sections 1814(c) and 1835(d)); hospitals and physicians outside of the U.S. (sections 1814(f) and 1862(a)(4)); and hospitals and SNFs of the Indian Health Service (section 1880 of the Act). Section 1877 of the Act sets forth limitations on referrals and payment for designated health services furnished by entities with which the referring physician (or an immediate family member of the referring physician) has a financial relationship.

Table 8.1 Stark and anti-kickback comparison

	Stark law	Anti-kickback
Definition	Prohibits a physician from referring patients covered by CMS entities to an entity where the physician has a financial relationship	Prohibits incentives or rewards for referrals or generation of federal healthcare program business
Encounter	From physicians	From anyone
Services defined	Designated health services	Any service
Federal healthcare programs	All	Medicare/medicaid

Marketing

The presence of continuing to meet the need of a community is the underlining goal of developing a referral network and offering healthcare. The resources available in the community and the appreciation for lead generation or consumer interest guide the strategy of the referral development. These marketing strategies include:

1. Print

    (a) Brochure
    (b) Mailers
    (c) Referral packet for patients
    (d) Referral packet for providers

2. Digital presence

    (a) Website
    (b) Driving traffic to the site

3. Social media

    (a) Twitter
    (b) Blogging

Oftentimes, a market analysis of the area is prudent, as development of a lead generation focus is contingent on understanding the mechanisms for the patient's access to healthcare. Notwithstanding, careful reanalysis of the mechanism is vital for molding the marketing plan.

Summary

Referral networks are a vital strategy for healthcare and strategy for creation of a pathway for patients to access healthcare efficiently and appropriately. Key components include an understanding of an integration among specialties, as well as relationship and network building. With careful planning, these networks will fuel patient-centric care.

References

1. Horst PK, Choo K, Bharucha N, et al. Graduates of orthopaedic residency training are increasingly subspecialized: a review of the American Board of Orthopaedic Surgery Part II Database. J Bone Joint Surg Am. 2015;97(10):869–75.
2. Pope JE, Ryan N, Carlson J, et al. Pain practice development and marketing in the digital age: a case study in an office-based interventional pain practice. International Neuromodulation Society Meeting, Poster Presentation, Montreal, Canada; 2015.
3. Quintner JL, Cohen ML, Buchanan D, et al. Pain medicine and its models: helping or hurting. Pain Med. 2008;9(7):824–34.
4. Pope JE, Deer TR, McRoberts WP. Intrathecal therapy: the burden of being positioned as a salvage therapy. Pain Med. 2015;16(10):2036–8.
5. Deer T, Caraway D, Wallace M. A definition of refractory pain to help determine suitability for device implantation. Neuromodulation. 2014;17(8):711–5. doi:10.1111/ner.12263. Noabstractavailable.
6. Healthcare Fraud Prevention and Enforcement Action Team (HEAT); Office of Inspector General; Comparison of the Anti-kickback statute and Stark Law.
7. Office of Inspector General, HHS. Medicare and state health care programs: fraud and abuse; electronic health records safe harbor under the anti-kickback statute. Final rule. Fed Regist. 2013;78(249):79201–20.
8. Taormina M. The Stark truth: what your physician clients should know about Stark Law and the Anti-Kickback Statute. J Health Care Finance. 2013;39(3):85–92.

Chapter 9
Integration of Specialties

Steven M. Falowski

Key Points

- Spinal cord stimulation (SCS) is a procedure that, in most cases, is considered minimally invasive, is performed as an outpatient same-day procedure, and has a very-low-risk profile.
- SCS has class I evidence of its superiority when placed against conventional medical management and against repeat spinal surgery.
- As a spine surgeon it is paramount to have a relationship with an interventional pain physician performing these procedures to foster the options for your patients or to offer the therapies in your practice.
- Those involved in the multidisciplinary approach range and span beyond primary care physicians, pain management physicians, and spine surgeons.

Introduction

The treatment of chronic pain can be very challenging. As a spine surgeon it is important to be able to treat your patients throughout their disease process. A radiographic and technically successful surgery does not always translate into the patient results that one desires. It is known that at least 30–40 % of spine surgery patients will develop post-laminectomy syndrome/failed back surgery syndrome (FBSS) [1, 2]. The literature supports that SCS can produce at least 50 % pain relief in 50–60 %

S.M. Falowski, M.D. (✉)
Neurosurgery, St. Luke's University Health Network,
701 Ostrum St, Suite 302, Bethlehem, PA 18017, USA
e-mail: sfalowski@gmail.com

© Springer International Publishing Switzerland 2016
S.M. Falowski, J.E. Pope (eds.), *Integrating Pain Treatment into Your Spine Practice*, DOI 10.1007/978-3-319-27796-7_9

of the implanted patients and reduce the use of more medications [1]. Proper follow-up care is necessary to ensure maintenance and success of the therapy. Of most importance in the literature is that there is class I evidence in multiple trials to demonstrate the efficacy of SCS [1, 3]. It has been compared against best medical management as well as surgery [1, 3].

As the treating spine surgeon it is important to be able to offer therapies to your patients when pain persists following surgery, or perhaps when pain is present without a surgical pathology. The ability to offer your patient options not only fosters the doctor–patient relationship, but also serves as an important treatment modality in this clearly defined subset of patients in a complex spine practice.

Multidisciplinary Approach

Most physicians will utilize a screening SCS trial prior to permanent implantation of the system. There are several factors that are important in being aware of these therapies and having access to them for your patients.

You will need to set up a proper referral network. This is determined by deciding whether you want to perform the therapies yourself or be willing to work with someone else who performs these therapies. Several models exist to integrate care among specialties and to deliver the appropriate care and treatment algorithm to your patients. As a spine surgeon, you can quickly become known for offering these advanced therapies, or at least fostering the appropriate pathway to obtain them.

These patients exist throughout the realm of medicine and are treated by multiple potential referring physicians. Patients usually are involved in a multidisciplinary setting and it is important to identify potential candidates throughout their course in traversing the medical field. The most common treating physicians include primary care and internal medicine physicians, neurologists, and pain physicians. As a spine surgeon in your community, you will likely receive many referrals for an evaluation for candidacy for spinal surgery, and in the majority of cases the patient will not be a candidate. Serendipitously, these patients may also be the same patients who would benefit from interventional pain therapies or neuromodulation. This leads to diversifying your offerings, developing a niche among spine surgeons, and creating a patient-centric referral network while also delivering more cases to your practice.

Another important aspect of any practice is building relationships with doctors in your referral network. This is most commonly the pain management specialist when considering a spinal surgery practice, but this should not overshadow the relationship with primary care, internal medicine, and neurologists who may also be involved in your referral network. Establishing relationships leads to your ultimate role in the treatment algorithm. It is important to realize that the role of the surgeon does not end with the surgical procedure, and that other specialties become involved in the treatment of these patients throughout their disease process and recovery.

Surgeons will commonly need to make decisions on whether patient's pain patterns can be improved with spinal surgery, and most importantly if surgery is the right path for the patient. Commonly, surgeons are concerned with having inappropriate surgical candidates in their clinic, but ultimately offering these therapies can increase your case volume as you consider these patients would have normally be turned away from your practice as not suitable for spinal surgery.

Earlier intervention in the appropriate patients leads to success in neuromodulation. These patients are receiving care among many specialties and identification of potential candidates throughout their treatment algorithm is of the utmost importance. Education, awareness, and relationships are paramount in delivering these therapies. Specific to surgeons, you have the ability to identify these patients early in the process and offer options which will alleviate their pain and prevent the potential long-term sequelae.

Summary

The benefits to your patients are clear in the setting of providing appropriate spine surgery. Literature suggests that up to 40 % of spinal patients will carry the diagnosis of FBSS [1, 2]. It is then crucial for spine surgeons to establish and maintain relationships with pain management specialists in the care of these patients. This role and relationship can be variable based on practice setup. It is also important to realize that this specific integration of the spine surgeon and pain management physician is only a part of the algorithm, as many specialties are involved in the care of patients who can benefit from neuromodulation. These can include primary care physicians, neurologists, rehabilitation physicians, and physical therapy.

Integration of pain therapies into your practice is crucial in appropriate care for your patients. If as a surgeon you choose not to perform these therapies, it is important that you know they are available and where patients will have access to them. Your patients will appreciate that you have offered them options and continued their care.

References

1. Kumar K, Taylor RS, Jacques L, et al. PROCESS study SCS vs CMM for FBSS. Pain. 2007;132(1–2):179–88.
2. Kumar K, et al. Spinal cord stimulation in treatment of chronic benign pain: challenges in treatment planning and present status, a 22-year experience. Neurosurgery. 2006;58(3):481–96. discussion 481–96.
3. North RB, Kidd DH, Farrokhi F, Piantadosi SA. SCS vs re-operation for FBSS*. Neurosurgery. 2005;56(1):98–106.

Chapter 10
Coding and Reimbursement for Spinal Cord Stimulation

Jason E. Pope and Steven M. Falowski

Key Points

- Formal education on coding and reimbursement is not performed currently in fellowship or residency programs.
- Incorrect coding and billing can result in repayment penalties or denials.
- Preauthorization is recommended for spinal cord stimulation.
- Local coverage determinations and national coverage determinations describe medical necessity for certain procedures.
- ICD codes describe diagnosis.
- CPT codes describe procedures.
- SCS coding and claim submission have undergone changes within the last few years.

Introduction

Capturing the clinical encounter is an important aspect of medicine that oftentimes is left to the provider to be self-taught while on the job. There is no formal billing didactic and the ACGME (Accreditation Counsel of Graduate Medical Education) or ABMS (American Board of Medical Specialties) does not

J.E. Pope, M.D., D.A.B.P.M., F.I.P.P. (✉)
Summit Pain Alliance, 392 Tesconi Court, Santa Rosa, CA 95401, USA
e-mail: popeje@me.com

S.M. Falowski, M.D.
Neurosurgery, St. Luke's University Health Network,
701 Ostrum St, Suite 302, Bethlehem, PA 18017, USA
e-mail: sfalowski@gmail.com

© Springer International Publishing Switzerland 2016
S.M. Falowski, J.E. Pope (eds.), *Integrating Pain Treatment into Your Spine Practice*, DOI 10.1007/978-3-319-27796-7_10

require proficiency prior to residency or fellowship completion. Despite this, CMS (Center for Medicare and Medicaid Services) requires accurate coding and billing for payment of services, as failure to do so in either direction would result in repayment penalties.

Coding and Billing

Historically, payments for medical encounters are dependent on National Coverage Determinations (NCD) and Local Coverage Determinations (LCD). These coverage determinations may vary and the reader is directed to their regional carrier. ICD-10 (international classification of diseases and health-related problems) is used to qualify the clinical scenario and disease being treated. CPT (current procedural terminology) codes are used to describe procedures employed to treat diseases. Therefore, for example once a patient is evaluated for spinal cord stimulation, the ICD-9 or ICD-10 description of the disease has to meet medical necessity from the NCD and LCD for the procedure (CPT code) to be reimbursed for payment. Further, two payments are typically administered for a given procedural service: a professional fee and a facility fee. Based on the site where service occurs, both fees can change. If this description sounds too simple, it is, as certified coders are typically employed in all practice types and sites of service. The fee schedules for the services provided are usually contracted between the provider and the insurance company. Accuracy and timeliness of supportive documentation are vital.

The site of service and professional fees dramatically vary based on the location of the procedure, with yearly updates. See the following determination 2015 for spinal cord stimulation (Fig. 10.1) [1].

Once a service is rendered, diagnosis codes (ICD-9 or ICD-10) and procedure codes (CPT) are assigned, and the claim is sent to the insurance carrier for consideration of payment, based on NCD and LCD of medical necessity. Oftentimes, qualifying the service will be needed. This is performed by assessing whether a treatment for a diagnosis, once submitted as a claim, meets medical necessity and the provider would receive payment. Providers can request these assessments as follows:

		Office (CF=$35.8228)				ASC			HOPD	
CPT	Description	Physician	Overhead	Total	Physician	Facility	ASC total	Physician	Facility	Total
63650	Implant neuroelectrodes (NA=National price is Not Available)	423.89	925.82	1,349.71	423.89	3,836.95	4,260.84	423.89	5,288.58	5712.47
63655	Implant neuroelectrodes (NA=National price is Not Available)	854.22			854.22	15,854.21	16,708.43	854.22	17,099.35	17953.57
63661	Remove spine eltrd perq aray	329.73	259.20	588.93	329.73	758.63	1,088.36	329.73	1,383.53	1713.26
63662	Remove spine eltrd plate	865.32			865.32	1,166.84	2,032.16	865.32	2,127.98	2993.30
63663	Remove spine eltrd perq aray	463.98	337.61	801.59	463.98	3,836.95	4,300.93	463.98	5,288.58	5752.56
63664	Remove spine eltrd plate	885.01	-	885.01	885.01	3,836.95	4,721.96	885.01	5,288.58	6173.59
63685	Implant neuroreceiver	377.35	-	377.35	377.35	20,806.60	21,183.95	377.35	26,152.16	26529.51
63688	Revise/remove neuroreceiver	381.28	-	381.28	381.28	1,166.84	1,548.12	381.28	2,127.98	2509.26

Fig. 10.1 Site of service fee schedule [1]

Predetermination

The coverage for payment of the service is predetermined before services are rendered and any deficiency of coverage by an insurance plan can be addressed prospectively, although it is not required.

Preauthorization

Preauthorization is a required process that allows a patient and providers the opportunity to determine coverage and procure an authorization or approval from a payor for a proposed treatment or service prior to performing the service. Unfortunately, preauthorization does not guarantee reimbursement.

Indications and Patient Selection for Spinal Cord Stimulation

Despite painstaking efforts [2–5] of these therapies to be positioned earlier in the algorithm than last resort, the NCD [6] for spinal cord stimulation (dorsal column stimulation) requires all these below conditions are met:

1. *The implantation of the stimulator is used only as a late resort (if not a last resort) for patients with chronic intractable pain.*
2. *With respect to item a, other treatment modalities (pharmacological, surgical, physical, or psychological therapies) have been tried and did not prove satisfactory, or are judged to be unsuitable or contraindicated for the given patient.*
3. *Patients have undergone careful screening, evaluation, and diagnosis by a multidisciplinary team prior to implantation. (Such screening must include psychological as well as physical evaluation.)*
4. *All the facilities, equipment, and professional and support personnel required for the proper diagnosis, treatment training, and follow-up of the patient (including that required to satisfy item c) must be available.*
5. *Demonstration of pain relief with a temporarily implanted electrode precedes permanent implantation.*

The indications for spinal cord stimulation, on-label, by the Food and Drug Administration (FDA) are neuropathic pain of the trunk or limbs.

The LCD for Spinal Cord Stimulation in Northern California, covered by Noridian [6, 7], is code L33489. Interesting components of the code are bolded.

The implantation of spinal cord stimulators (SCS) may be covered as therapies for the relief of chronic intractable pain. SCS is best suited for neuropathic pain but may have some limited value in other types of nociceptive severe, intractable pain. Therapy consists of a short trial with a percutaneous implantation of neurostimulator electrode(s) in the epidural space for assessing a patient's suitability for ongoing treatment with a permanent surgically implanted nerve stimulator. Performance and documentation of an effective trial is a prerequisite for permanent nerve stimulation.

Selection of patients for implantation of spinal cord stimulators is critical to success of this therapy. SCS therapy should be considered as a late (if not last) resort after more conservative attempts such as medications, physical therapy, surgery, psychological therapy, or other modalities have been tried.

Patients must have undergone careful screening, evaluation, and diagnosis by a multidisciplinary team prior to implantation. (Such screening must include psychological as well as physical evaluation.) Documentation of the history and careful screening must be available in the patient chart if requested. Patients being selected for a trial

Must not have active substance abuse issues.
Must undergo proper patient education, discussion, and disclosure including an extensive discussion of the risks and benefits of this therapy.
Must undergo appropriate psychological screening.

Many experts recommend that the temporary neurostimulator be placed in an ASC or outpatient hospital setting. However, the temporary neurostimulator trial can be done in an office setting if all the sterility, equipment, professional training, and support personnel required for the proper surgery and follow-up of the patient are available. Permanent neurostimulators must be placed in an ASC or hospital. Physicians performing SCS trials in the office setting must have like privileges at a local hospital or ASC, or the providers must be subspecialty boarded in Pain Medicine by the American Board of Anesthesiology.

It is preferable that physicians performing the SCS trial will also perform the permanent implant. If the physician implanting the trial neurostimulator does not or cannot implant the permanent neurostimulator, the patient should be informed of this in writing and given the name of the referral surgeon who will implant the permanent neurostimulator(s).

It is expected that accurate patient selection will lead to most patients going on to receive permanent implants. Only patients who experience a positive response to a trial should proceed to a permanent implantation. All trials which proceed to permanent implant must have adequate documentation in the chart to support that decision. A successful trial should be associated with at least a 50 % reduction of target pain, or 50 % reduction of analgesic medications, and show some element of functional improvement. (Patients with reflex sympathetic dystrophy may show lower levels of improvement since it takes longer periods for improvement than the typical 1–2-week trial.) Physician judgment and experience will also be taken into account.

Physicians with a low trial-to-permanent implant ratio (less than 50 %) will be subject to post-payment review and may be asked to submit documentation as to the patient selection criteria, the radiologic imaging demonstrating proper lead placement, and the medical necessity of the trials. Failure to provide this documentation will be cause for post-payment denial and recoupment of reimbursement. It is understood that all patients may not have a favorable result of the trial implant; but careful selection should find the most appropriate patients.

Table 10.1 Spinal cord simulation disease indications

Ideal candidates
CRPS
Ischemic pain
Neuropathy (diabetes or metabolic disorder)
Cervical or lumbar persistent radiculopathy!
"Failed surgery syndrome"
Moderate candidates
Axial pain
Truncal pain
Low candidates
Central pain
Spinal cord or brain injury neuropathic pain
Phantom pain
Avulsion injury

Noridian will reimburse for placement of a maximum of 2 leads or 16 "contacts," and for 2 SCS trials per anatomic spinal region per patient per lifetime.

If a trial fails, a repeat trial is not appropriate unless there are extenuating circumstances that lead to trial failure. Appropriate medical documentation to support a repeat trial can be sent on appeal.

In the description of the LCD, there is no classification of what diagnosis warrants SCS based on medical necessity. Commonly, SCS is approved for indication outlined in Table 10.1 [Deer/Pope Atlas]. It should be noted that Medicare requires a primary and secondary diagnosis for the placement of spinal cord stimulators (Table 10.2). Perhaps the most common is a primary code of Chronic Pain syndrome, with a secondary code that may include Post Laminectomy syndrome, Lumbar radiculopathy, or CRPS.

CPT Codes for Spinal Cord Stimulation

Please refer to Table 10.3 regarding CPT codes for the use in spinal cord stimulation. General rules are as follows: The codes are determined based on the type of lead, not the reason for placement (for the trial or the permanent). During the trial phase, the lead removal is implied in the original code and an explant code is not used. In addition, initial programming is implied in the original code. Of note, open surgical trial codes do not include the explant or the programming. Most often, orthopedic and neurosurgeons engage in the implant or revision phase of the procedure. This includes CPT codes for the internal pulse generator (IPG) and the revision procedure, respectively. The pulse generator can be either a rechargeable or a non-rechargeable system; although the coding is the same (63685), overall the device costs for the facility are different (rechargeable batteries are more expensive than the primary cell devices). When laminectomy leads are placed, the code 63685 is used. When leads are placed in an area of an existing laminectomy site, the code 63664 is utilized.

Table 10.2 Typical ICD-10 diagnosis codes for spinal cord stimulation

Chronic pain disorders			
	338.0	Central pain syndrome	
	338.29	Other chronic pain	
	338.4	Chronic pain syndrome	
CRPS			
	337.21	CRPS type I of the upper limb	
	337.22	CRPS type I of the lower limb	
	354.4	CRPS type II of the upper extremity	
	355.71	CRPS type II of the lower extremity	
Spinal diagnosis			
	322.2	Arachnoiditis, chronic	
	322.9	Arachnoiditis, other	
	722.10	Lumbar radiculitis due to herniated disc	
	722.52	Radiculitis due to degenerative disc disease, lumbar	
	722.83	Post-laminectomy syndrome, lumbar	
	722.81	Post-laminectomy syndrome, cervical	
	723.4	Radicular syndrome of upper limbs (not due to disc herniation or degeneration)	
	724.4	Radicular syndrome of the lower limbs (not due to herniation or degeneration)	
Peripheral neuropathy	354.9	Peripheral neuropathy of the upper limb	
	255.8	Peripheral neuropathy of the lower limb	
Abdominal	338.29	Chronic abdominal pain	

Table 10.3 CPT codes for SCS

63650	Trial spinal cord stimulation
63655	Laminectomy spinal cord stimulation implant
63650	Percutaneous spinal cord stimulation implant
63685	Insertion spinal cord stimulator internal pulse generator (IPG)
63663	Revising a percutaneous lead with placemat in the same location
63664	Revising a laminectomy lead with placement in the same location

Coding Examples [8, 9]

Percutaneous Trial with separate Percutaneous Permanent Implantation

Trial Placement (including lead removal and programming): 63650
Percutaneous Permanent Placement: 63650, 63685(IPG), 95972(Programming)

Percutaneous Trial with direct conversion to Percutaneous Permanent Implantation

First Procedure with Trial Placement and Tunneled Extensions (including lead removal and programming): 63650
Second Procedure with Permanent Placement: 63685

Percutaneous Trial with Surgical Paddle Permanent Implantation

Trial Placement (including lead removal and programming): 63650
Permanent Placement: 63655 (Paddle), 63685 (IPG), 95972 (Programming)

Open Surgical Trial with Direct conversion to Paddle Permanent Implantation

First Procedure with Lead Placement and Tunneled Extensions: 63655, 95972
Second Procedure if removal for failed trial: 63662 (Removal Paddle)
Second Procedure if permanent placement: 63664 (Revision of paddle), 63685, 95972

It should be noted that 63664 can only be used if significant work is involved in exposing or repositioning the previously placed lead.

Summary

Coding and billing are key components to reimbursement and a mindful approach of national and local coverage determinations, along with an appreciation for diagnosis and procedure codes, will ensure success and allow patients access to these important treatment modalities. Changes in how these devices are reimbursed regarding the site of service and the number of contacts have created a more patient-centered approach to neuromodulation, focused on safety and outcomes.

References

1. American Society of Interventional Pain Physicians®. Comparison of 2015 Medicare fee schedule in three settings. https://www.asipp.org/documents/20153SettingsComparison.pdf. Accessed 30 Oct 2015.
2. Pope JE, Deer TR, McRoberts WP. Intrathecal therapy: the burden of being positioned as a salvage therapy. Pain Med. 2015;16(10):2036–8.
3. Deer T, Caraway D, Wallace M. A definition of refractory pain to help determine suitability for device implantation. Neuromodulation. 2014;17(8):711–5. doi:10.1111/ner.12263.Noabstract available.
4. Poree L, Krames E, Pope J, et al. Spinal cord stimulation as treatment for complex regional pain syndrome should be considered earlier than last resort therapy. Neuromodulation. 2013;16(2):125–41.
5. Kumar K, Toth C, Nath RK, Laing P. Epidural spinal cord stimulation for treatment of chronic pain—some predictors of success. A 15 year experience. Surg Neurol. 1998;50(2):110–20.
6. Centers for Medicare & Medicaid Services. National Coverage Determination (NCD) for Electrical Nerve Stimulators (160.7). Updated: 8/7/1995. https://www.cms.gov/medicare-coverage-database/details/ncd-details.aspx?NCDId=240&ncdver=1&DocID=160.7&SearchType=Advanced&bc=IAAAABAAAAAA&. Accessed 30 Oct 2015.

7. Centers for Medicare & Medicaid Services. Local Coverage Determination (LCD): spinal cord stimulators for chronic pain (L33489). Updated: 9/1/2014. http://www.cms.gov/medicare-coverage-database/details/lcd-details.aspx?LCDId=33489&ContrId=364&ver=12&ContrVer=1&CntrctrSelected=364*1&Cntrctr=364&name=&DocType=Active&s=66&bc=AggAAAIAAAAAAA%3d%3d&. Accessed 30 Oct 2015.
8. Medtronic. Neurostimulation therapy for chronic pain— trunk and/or limbs commonly billed codes. Updated: January 2015. http://professional.medtronic.com/wcm/groups/mdtcom_sg/@mdt/@neuro/documents/documents/scs-codes.pdf. Accessed 30 Oct 2015.
9. Medtronic. Spinal cord stimulation for chronic pain — trunk and/or limbs clarifications on CPT coding for SCS leads. Updated: 7/11/2011. http://professional.medtronic.com/wcm/groups/mdt-com_sg/@mdt/@neuro/documents/documents/scs_lead_coding_summary_2011_0.pdf. Accessed 30 Oct 2015.

Part III
Pain Management Therapies

Chapter 11
Medications Used for the Treatment of Back Pain

Jonathan D. Carlson, Joshua Peloquin, and Steven M. Falowski

Key Points

- Physicians are encouraged to adhere to a pain management algorithm with the primary driver being utilization of the full spectrum of minimally invasive and invasive surgical techniques, physical medicine, and pain medications to ameliorate the patient's pain symptoms.
- **Nonsteroidal anti-inflammatory drugs (NSAIDs) and acetaminophen**: Initial therapy for back pain. Acetaminophen dose should not exceed 2 g/day.
- **Muscle relaxants**: When prescribed concurrently with NSAIDS, their use appears to be additive and patients report greater pain relief.
- **Antiepileptics**: Are especially beneficial to patients suffering from neuropathic pain. This class of medications must be titrated up slowly to effective doses. It is important to remember that antiepileptic medications often do not impact pain immediately and must be used for weeks to months before effects are optimized.
- **Antidepressants**: Many chronic pain patients suffer from depression. Depression can hinder the effectiveness of other pain management modalities. Tricyclic antidepressants also appear to have a direct effect on neuropathic pain.

J.D. Carlson, M.D. (✉)
Interventional Pain, Pain Doctor, LLC, Midwestern Medical School,
18555 N. 79th Ave., D101, Glendale, AZ 85308, USA
e-mail: jcarlsonmd@gmail.com

J. Peloquin, D.O.
Midwestern Medical School, Internal Medicine Intern,
431 Cartier Pl, Placentia, CA 92870, USA
e-mail: joshua.peloquin@gmail.com

S.M. Falowski, M.D.
Neurosurgery, St. Luke's University Health Network,
701 Ostrum St, Suite 302, Bethlehem, PA 18017, USA
e-mail: sfalowski@gmail.com

© Springer International Publishing Switzerland 2016   99
S.M. Falowski, J.E. Pope (eds.), *Integrating Pain Treatment into Your Spine Practice*, DOI 10.1007/978-3-319-27796-7_11

- **Opioids**: Potent pain medication; should only be prescribed after NSAIDS and other treatments have failed including interventional pain procedures. Their use also should not obviate the need to assess other pain management modalities such as physical therapy, pain procedures, weight loss regimen, and home exercise therapy. When the decision is made to prescribe opioids for chronic nonmalignant pain, adhering to the recommended best practices is often considered the "Standard of Care" by most State Medical Boards.

Introduction

Both patients and physicians should fully engage in the use of the less invasive alternatives available for chronic pain treatment prior to use of more invasive surgical procedures. These alternative treatments include medications such as NSAIDs, steroid burst, muscle relaxants, antidepressants and antiepileptics, and opioids. Acupuncture, chiropractic care, and physical therapy are also found to be effective treatments to aid the reduction of a patient's chronic pain. Minimally invasive procedures such as epidural steroid injections, peripheral nerve blocks, radiofrequency ablation, spinal stimulation, and intrathecal medication pumps should also be considered early in the treatment algorithm. Although there are many different methods for treating chronic pain, this chapter will primarily focus on the classic pain medications for the treatment of acute and chronic back pain.

NSAIDs and Acetaminophen for Pain Management of Back Pain

When the onset of back pain first occurs, the guidelines for treatment from the American Pain Society, American Academy of Pain Management, and American College of Physicians state that patients should begin initial treatment with first line medications such as acetaminophen and NSAIDs [1]. When utilizing acetaminophen, doses should not exceed 2 g/day in patients without evidence of liver disease. When a physician is administering any medications to patients, including first line medications such as acetaminophen and NSAIDs, it is imperative to match up a medications side effect profile with patient's current comorbidities. Clearly, hepatic and renal failure would preclude use of such agents, respectively. NSAIDS, such as ketoprofen and nabumetone, are good options for treating pain patients. Nabumatome is found to have a better gastrointestinal side effect profile then many other NSAIDS [2] and is a good choice for patients suffering from GERD or who have a history of ulcers. It also has short-term gastroprotective qualities many other nonselective NSAIDS do not possess and is effective when used in short durations. A meta-analysis comparing ketoprofen, ibuprofen, and diclofenac showed ketoprofen to have statistically significant superiority when compared to other NSAIDs [3]. Recently, first-line treatments such as NSAIDs and acetaminophen have decreased in popularity among prescribing doctors in the treatment of pain. To analyze the decline in NSAID and acetaminophen use by prescribing physicians, a study was conducted by John N. Mafi et al. from the National Ambulatory Medical Care Survey and the National Hospital Ambulatory Medical Care Survey. The study cataloged nearly 24,000 visits for spine disorders and is widely thought to be a representative sample of the approximately 440 million patient visits caused by chronic pain in 2013. Data within the study showed the use of NSAIDs and acetaminophen decreased between 2000 and 2010 (from 37 to 29 %). The use of opioid medications increased (from 19 to 29 %) over the same time span [4].

Opioids for Pain Management

This switch must be approached with care and consideration by the prescribing provider. The medical evidence-based application of opioids for the treatment of chronic noncancer pain is lacking supportive randomized controlled trials. Scant evidence and the marked rise of opioid-related deaths in the USA, necessitated the development of best practices with prescribing chronic opioids for noncancer pain. As a cautionary note, many state medical boards consider these best practices recommendations to be the "Standard of Care." Several physicians have been censured and/or had their medical licenses revoked when there has been a consistent pattern with failure to comply linked to patient deaths from opioid overdose (Table 11.1).

Table 11.1 Opioid conversions

1. Calculate total mg dose taken in past 24-h.
2. Determine equi-analgesic dose (table).
3. If pain is controlled on current opioid, reduce the new opioid daily dose by 30–50 % to account for cross-tolerance.
4. If inpatient with proper monitoring, methodically titrate to achieve analgesic effect during first 24 h and/or consider patient controlled analgesia (PCA)
5. Monitor for adverse events and effectiveness.

Buprenorphine (IM/IV): 0.4 mg	Meperidine (IV/IM/SC): 75 mg
Butorphanol (IM/IV): 2.0 mg	Meperidine (PO): 300 mg
Codeine (IM/IV): 120 mg	Methadone (acute IV): 5.0 mg
Codeine (PO): 200 mg	Methadone (acute PO): 10 mg
Fentanyl (IM/IV): 0.1 mg	Morphine (IV/IM/SC): 10 mg
Fentanyl (Transdermal): 0.2 mg	Morphine (acute PO): 60 mg
Hydrocodone (PO): 30 mg	Morphine (chronic PO): 30 mg
Hydromorphone (IV/IM/SC): 1.5 mg	Oxycodone (PO): 20 mg
Hydromorphone (PO): 7.5 mg	Oxymorphone (IV/IM/SC): 1.0 mg
	Oxymorphone (PO): 10 mg

Disclaimer: It should be noted that these conversions are not definitive and should only be used as a guide. Vigilance with individual patient application of opioids conversions is still at the sole discretion of the prescribing provider

Chronic Opioid Prescribing Best Practices to Mitigate Opioid Overdose [5]
1. Confirmation of pathology which warrants opioids via a thorough history and physical exam as well as appropriate diagnostic testing.
2. Exhaust non-opioid based medications when possible.
3. Review of medical records to rule out potential contraindications (suicide, diversion, illicit drug use, addiction, noncompliance, lack of legitimate diagnosis, etc.)
4. Implement patient–physician opioid agreement.
5. Screen for opioid diversion: routine urine/oral drug screening, review of online state-controlled prescription monitoring program (if available) to assess if receiving opioids from several different providers (rule out "doctor shopping" or "double dipping"), rule out multiple early refill requests, random pill counts, etc.

Opioid medications should only be used for the treatment of pain when the severity of the pain warrants it and with confirmed pathology. Typically, this potent medication should only be considered when the patient's pain is affecting their activities of daily living and function, and when multiple non-opioid pain medications have failed to adequately control the patient's pain. Visual Analogue Scale (VAS) pain scores alone can be misleading. Each patient's physiological response to opioid treatments will be unique and a tailored approach should be implemented to reduce the possibility of over-medicating. When treatment is initiated, it should be required by the physician that the patient agrees to abide by a patient–physician opioid agreement. This agreement specifies the patient is not to consume any alcohol, marijuana, or other illegal substances. Patients must also agree to undergo periodic and unscheduled urine drug screens (UDS) to test for illegal substance abuse as well as to monitor if the prescribed medication is being utilized. UDS are a simple test that can screen for metabolites of commonly abused substances and medications. An example of this is patients who use heroin in conjunction with prescribed opioids will test positive for 6-monoacetylmorphine (6-MAM) for approximately 12 h after substance abuse occurs (Fig. 11.1). Beyond this 12 h window only morphine will be present in the patients UDS. The following image illustrates the metabolites of heroin and its eventual metabolism to morphine in the body. Tramadol, methadone, and ketamine are also very effective pain management medications that have both opioid receptor activity and NMDA receptor activities. Methadone and ketamine have very complex pharmacodynamics and pharmacokinetics with a high propensity for overdose potential; thus, they are often reserved for proficient pain specialists.

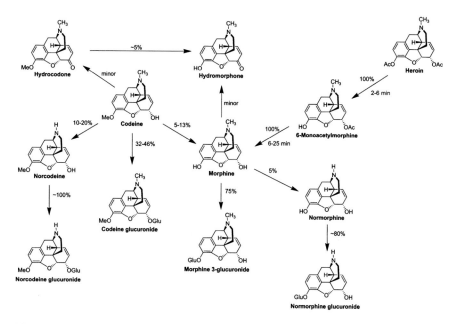

Fig. 11.1 Morphine-based metabolites

Tailoring Opioid Doses for Patient-Specific Needs

A tailored approach requires the potency and dose of opioids to be increased incrementally as pain symptoms and patient comorbidities dictate.

Contraindications for Opioids
- Lack of appropriate pathology
- Severe respiratory instability
- Severe psychiatric instability or suicide risk
- Unaddressed or recent substance use disorder
- Severe opioid allergy/side effects
- Co-administration of drugs capable of inducing life-threatening interactions.
- Inappropriate use of medication (providing medication to others, concurrent alcohol use, concurrent or illegal substance use

For cases of mild pain, the initial regimen should be a nonsteroidal anti-inflammatory drug (NSAIDs) or acetaminophen. For moderate levels of pain, an opioid receptor agonist such as tramadol, hydrocodone, or oxycodone can be paired alongside with NSAIDs or acetaminophen when deemed appropriate. In cases of severe pain, a higher potency opioid receptor agonist such as morphine, hydromorphone, oxymorphone, methadone, or fentanyl may be considered for use. DNA testing appears to be a promising new method of tailored prescribing. Genetic testing can assist a physician in determining which opioids are most appropriate for a specific patient. Genetic sampling of saliva is easily done during the initial patient evaluation.

Several of the opioids listed above can be modified to increase the duration of their effectiveness. These modified opioids are typically found in forms such as extended-release tablets. These long-acting opioid treatments should only be given to patients who are considered to have high opioid tolerance and when treatment with short-acting opioids alone provides suboptimal pain relief. Patients who fall into this category of treatment must be closely monitored for adverse effects. Extended-release tablets should never be used to treat acute or postoperative pain, or opioid-naive patients. Patients should be warned to never split extended-release pills into partial doses or crush medications. Such actions can cause immediate release of 12–24 h amount of dosing, thus causing adverse effects such as respiratory depression and overdose/death.

When physicians are developing a tailored approach for patient care, it is important to note opioid medications, while powerful in the treatment of pain, are only one variable in the treatment of a patient's pain. The use of opioids should not delay early implementation of other therapies and modalities such as exercise and physical therapy when medically indicated. A multimodal approach paired with supplementation of opioids to alleviate pain is common practice. Vigilant attentiveness to ruling out diversion is paramount and cannot be over emphasized. Careful attention should be placed on avoiding long-term opioid use when other interventions have not been exhausted including interventional procedures.

Proper Rotation and Conversion of Opioids for Ongoing Pain Management

As treatment continues, chronic pain patients may develop a tolerance to the opioid medications they are currently prescribed. Opioid medication rotation can be considered by the physician if this occurs. The proper conversion dosages for opioid rotation can be calculated with the following table (Table 11.1).

Muscle Relaxants

Muscle relaxants such as cyclobenzaprine (Flexeril) and methocarbamol (Robaxin) are found to be effective supplements for patients who are currently treating lower back pain with NSAIDs or acetaminophen. Evidence suggests that when taken in tandem with NSAIDs or acetaminophen, muscle relaxants are thought to provide more effective short-term pain relief compared to NSAIDs and acetaminophen alone. It is estimated 35 % of patients who visit their primary care physician for the treatment of low back pain are prescribed muscle relaxants. In 2003, Tulder et al. performed a Cochrane review of the efficacy of muscle relaxants and low back pain. The study was comprised of 30 randomized double-blinded trials. The trials provided evidence to support the effectiveness of muscle relaxants as an effective treatment of both acute and chronic lower back pain [6]. The effectiveness and acceptance of muscle relaxants for chronic pain is not without controversy.

The controversy lies in the side effect profile of most muscle relaxants. Muscle relaxant side effects are numerous with the most common being sedation, drowsiness, headache, blurred vision, nausea, vomiting, and increased probability of falls in the geriatric population. Muscle relaxants such as Carisoprodol (Soma) and Diazepam (Valium) have also been found to have a high potential for abuse and dependency among patients. There is a synergistic effect when either of these two relaxants is combined with opioids that could lead to respiratory depression/apnea and death.

The most commonly used muscle relaxants include cyclobenzaprine (Flexeril), methocarbamol (Robaxin), baclofen, tizanidine (Zanaflex), and carisoprodol (Soma). Carisoprodol (Soma), although an effective muscle relaxant, should be avoided as a chronic treatment option due to its active metabolite meprobamate, which is a central acting tranquilizer. Meprobamate is highly addictive and potentially deadly. Because of its addictive qualities, it is often difficult for physicians to wean patients off of carisoprodol (Soma). Carisoprodol (Soma) usage has been the culprit for several patient deaths due to overmedication and the global medical community has taken note. In 2007, it was removed from the market in Sweden and in 2008, the country of Norway followed suit. Currently, the European Union has recommended the removal of marketing for carisoprodol to discourage its use.

Neuropathic Pain and Low Back Pain

Antidepressants and antiepileptics are typically used to treat patients who are suffering from neuropathic pain. Tricyclic antidepressants such as amitriptyline or nortriptyline, and antiepileptics such as gabapentin (Neurontin or Gralise), pregabalin (Lyrica) and topiramate are commonly utilized. A meta-analysis on the effects of antidepressant treatment on chronic back pain was done in 2003 by Salerno S et al. Their analysis indicated that patients who received antidepressant therapy for chronic back pain experienced a reduction in their chronic pain levels in comparison to the placebo group. The study also unveiled a small, but nonsignificant trend in patients who received the antidepressant treatments had improved function in their activities of daily living and in their daily quality of life [7, 8].

Patients who are prescribed antidepressants are placed at risk for several adverse symptoms, the most common being drowsiness, dry mouth, and dizziness. These side effects paired with antidepressants minimal upside for pain relief rule them out as a first-line treatment for primary chronic back pain [9]. However, depression is common in patients with chronic pain, and clinicians should assess and treat depression accordingly. The chronic pain many patients experience is often alleviated once their depressive symptoms are abated. Antidepressants such as the tricyclics are also found to be beneficial for treating patients suffering from neuropathic pain and insomnia.

Antiepileptics Used in Treatment of Radicular and Non-radicular Back Pain

Antiepileptic medications such as gabapentin, pregabalin, and topiramate appear to have a positive affect on patients suffering from radicular back pain. All three of these medications must be titrated up in order to reach the appropriate dose for each patient.

Example of Pregabalin Titration
- Initial: 75 mg PO Q 12H
- Week 2: 150 mg PO Q 12H
- Week 3: 300 mg PO Q 12H

It is important to closely follow the patient during the titration phase; monitoring for both serious and less consequential side effects. The serious side effects caused by antiepileptic medications include suicidal ideation, blurred vision, altered mental status, and decreased coordination. Less consequential side effects include dizziness, somnolence, and fatigue.

For the treatment of non-radicular pain topiramate appears to be moderately superior to gabapentin and is often the medication of choice for prescribing physicians. It should be noted that topiramate can have deleterious effects on fetal development and appropriate monitoring for pregnancy should always be done. Gabapentin can be utilized as a medication for patients who are suffering from spinal stenosis and who are already prescribed a pain medication regimen containing NSAIDs and exercise therapy. When gabapentin is added to a patient's pain medication regimen and titrated up to 2400 mg/day it appears to be more effective in mitigating the patient's pain symptoms than NSAIDS and exercise therapy alone [10]. It is imperative for both the patient and prescribing physician to understand the immediate effects of these medications are limited. They can take weeks to months to reach their full effectiveness and adequate time should be allotted to achieve its optimal effect.

Summary

When considering treatments for chronic pain it is important for patients and physicians to consider all the treatments at their disposal before deciding on a plan. Physicians should treat the patient in a stepwise fashion starting with least invasive treatment with the lowest chances of side effects. This often times includes acetaminophen, NSAIDS, and physical therapy. As a first step up in the treatment of back pain, muscle relaxants, such as methocarbamol (Robaxin) or cyclobenzaprine (Flexeril), may be considered. When attempts to mitigate a patient's pain with NSAIDS, acetaminophen, muscle relaxants, and physical therapy have failed, and the patient has confirmed pathology, short-acting opioids may be considered. It is essential to start with the lowest dose and least potent opioid that may potentially alleviate the pain. Escalation of opioids should be executed slowly and only after careful consideration of other options. DEA evaluation of iatrogenic overdose and death from opioids has been linked with prescribing too high of an initial dose and/ or too rapid of an escalation with the opioid medication [5, 11].

If the patient is thought to suffer from neuropathic pain, antiepileptics such as gabapentin, pregabalin, and topiramate can be utilized. It is key for the patient as well as the prescriber to remember these medications must be titrated to effective levels and relief may take weeks to month to be fully appreciated. Tricyclic antidepressants such as amitriptyline or nortriptyline also play an important role in pain management. The mechanisms in which they work are not yet fully understood but their benefits make them a key component worthy of consideration when physicians are assessing the root of a patient's chronic back pain. Symptoms of depression are often found in chronic pain patients and it is thought to hinder the effectiveness of other pain management when left untreated. As a result, the treatment of depression, both with behavioral therapy and pharmaceutically, is often an integral piece of the pain treatment algorithm. This should not be discounted or overlooked by the treating physicians.

Effective pain management is an intricate algorithm comprised of multiple treatment techniques. While medications are an important piece of the pain management algorithm, it is only one variable among many which must be assessed when treating a patient's pain. It is imperative that the primary care provider, complementary medical staff, pain specialist, and surgeon work together to build a comprehensive pain management plan for each patient. This encompassing strategy will provide the most adequate and thorough treatment available to patients for chronic back pain.

References

1. Chou R, Qaseem A, Snow V, et al. Diagnosis and treatment of low back pain: a joint clinical practice guideline from the American College of Physicians and the American Pain Society. Ann Intern Med. 2007;147:478.
2. Peterson K, McDonagh M, Thakurta S, et al. Drug class reviews. Portland, OR: Oregon Health & Science University; 2010.
3. Sarzi-Puttini P, Atzeni F, Lanata L, et al. Efficacy of ketoprofen vs. ibuprofen and diclofenac: a systematic review of the literature and meta-analysis. Clin Exp Rheumatol. 2013;31(5):731–8. Epub 2013 May 17.
4. Mafi JN, McCarthy EP, Davis RB, et al. Worsening trends in the management and treatment of back pain. JAMA Intern Med. 2013;173:1573.

5. Mardian A, Patel T, Derksen D, Carlson J, et al. Arizona opioid prescribing guidelines. www. azdhs.gov/clinicians/documents/clinical-guidelines-recommendations/prescribing-guidelines/141121-opiod.pdf
6. van Tulder MW, Touray T, Furlan AD, et al. Muscle relaxants for nonspecific low back pain: a systematic review within the framework of the cochrane collaboration. Spine (Phila Pa 1976). 2003;28:1978.
7. Salerno SM, Browning R, Jackson JL. The effect of antidepressant treatment on chronic back pain: a meta-analysis. Arch Intern Med. 2002;162:19.
8. Staiger TO, Gaster B, Sullivan MD, et al. Systematic review of antidepressants in the treatment of chronic low back pain. Spine (Phila Pa 1976). 2003;28:2540.
9. Chou R, Huffman L. Medications for acute and chronic low back pain: a review of the evidence for an American Pain Society/American College of Physicians clinical practice guideline. Ann Intern Med. 2007;147(7):505–14.
10. Yaksi A, Ozgönenel L, Ozgönenel B. The efficiency of gabapentin therapy in patients with lumbar spinal stenosis. Spine (Phila Pa 1976). 2007;32:939.
11. Manchikanti L, Abdi S, Atluri S, et al. American Society of Interventional Pain Physicians (ASIPP) guidelines for responsible opioid prescribing in chronic non-cancer pain: Part 1—evidence assessment. Pain Physician. 2012;15(3 Suppl):S1–65.

Chapter 12
Interventional Procedures

Daniel A. Fung and Timothy T. Davis

Key Points

- Interventional procedures should be considered after conservative treatments (medications, therapy, activity modification) have failed and before surgical intervention.
- Physicians should be familiar with all medicare guidelines which have outlined specific criteria that must be accurately documented prior to proceeding with any interventional procedure.
- Trigger point injections are considered medically necessary when there is a regional muscular pain complaint with a palpable taut band in an accessible muscle and all conservative treatments have failed and been documented.
- Targeted medial branch blocks or intra-articular injections of the zygapophyseal joints (facet joints, z-joints) with local anesthetic are indicated when a diagnosis of cervical, thoracic, or lumbar spondylosis is established and correlated with regional pain in the respective area.
- Epidural injections are indicated in the cases of radicular pain that has failed all conservative treatments.
- SI joint injections will be considered medically necessary when an injection is given with imaging confirmation for diagnostic or therapeutic purposes after conservative management has failed.
- Discography is considered medically necessary for evaluation of disc pathology in persons with persistent, severe low back pain and abnormal interspaces on MRI, where other diagnostic tests have failed to reveal clear confirmation of a suspected disc as the source of pain and surgical intervention is being considered.

D.A. Fung, M.D. (✉) • T.T. Davis, M.D.
Orthopedic Pain Specialists, 2428 Santa Monica Blvd., Suite 208, Santa Monica, CA 90404, USA
e-mail: dfung@orthopaindocs.com; tdavis@orthopaindocs.com

© Springer International Publishing Switzerland 2016
S.M. Falowski, J.E. Pope (eds.), *Integrating Pain Treatment into Your Spine Practice*, DOI 10.1007/978-3-319-27796-7_12

Introduction

Minimally invasive interventional procedures should be considered when conservative modalities have failed to provide adequate relief. Selection of the proper interventional treatment is predicated on the accurate identification of a pain generator. There is no substitute for a thorough history and physical exam. Imaging should be used as a supportive tool to confirm the suspected diagnosis. The future of interventional pain medicine depends on a mindful and conservative application of procedures, based on published outcome data. There is no place in the near or long term for the "shot-gun" approach to identifying and treating sources of pain.

Medicare guidelines have outlined diagnosis-specific criteria that must be accurately documented prior to proceeding with any interventional pain therapy. Each interventional procedure is diagnosis specific and certain criteria must be met in order to validate a diagnosis. These diagnosis criteria are separated into "major" and "minor" criteria which consist of subjective complaints and objective findings. The authors recommend a review and full comprehensive understanding of the Medicare Coverage Database as it applies to each interventional procedure that is planned in practice [1].

This chapter provides a comprehensive review of the most common interventional procedures and discusses "evidence-based indications" with an overview of the proper execution of each type of procedure.

Trigger Point Injections

Myofascial trigger points are "small, circumscribed, hyperirritable foci in muscles and fascia, often found with a firm or taut band of skeletal muscle" [1]. When pressure is applied over the trigger point, local tenderness and occasionally radiating pain are elicited. Pressure or needle entry into the trigger point injections can sometimes elicit a local "twitch response" when the tense muscle involuntarily contracts.

Indications and Rationale

Trigger point injections are indicated when a diagnosis of myofascial pain syndrome is established as the source of a patient's pain. Direct pressure over the trigger point should reproduce the patient's pain and commonly associated radiating pattern.

Trigger point injections are considered medically necessary when there is a regional muscular pain complaint with a palpable taut band in an accessible muscle. All failed conservative treatments including therapy, medications, and activity modification must be documented. There must be exquisite spot tenderness at one point along the length of the taut band with some degree of restricted range of motion and pain or altered sensation in an expected distribution. The pain must be reproducible by pressure over the tender spot or a local twitch response or resolution of pain by stretching or injection [1].

Studies have shown a direct relationship between trigger point injections and improved pain, range of motion, and quality of life. In a randomized controlled trial Ay et al. showed that trigger point injections lead to statistically significant improvements in pain, range of motion, and depression scores with both local anesthetic injection and dry needling of trigger points [2].

Technique

Trigger points are identified by palpation over the painful muscle, a taut band of muscle is usually felt, and reproduction of the patient's pain is produced. Needle placement into the trigger point is typically performed in the office under the physician's knowledge of anatomy without specific equipment for guidance; however electromyography or nerve stimulation can be used to confirm placement and ultrasound can be used to visualize intramuscular placement [3]. When the needle is in place, medication (typically an anesthetic and a small amount of corticosteroid) is injected or dry needling can be performed. Directing and repositioning the needle in multiple planes within a trigger point area may help in further mechanical breakdown of the taut band. Some advocate the use of other injectates in trigger point injections such as botulinum toxin, prolotherapy, or platelet-rich plasma (PRP) which further treat the patient's pain through their individual healing mechanisms.

Paravertebral Facet Joint Block and Facet Joint Denervation

Targeted medial branch blocks or intra-articular injections of the zygapophyseal joints (facet joints, z-joints) with local anesthetic are indicated when a diagnosis of cervical, thoracic, or lumbar spondylosis is established and correlated with regional pain in the respective area. For coding purposes, "an injection may be placed in the facet joint itself or around the medial branch nerve innervating the joint" [1]. Diagnostic facet blocks must provide at least 80 % relief of an individual's usual and customary pain, in order to justify proceeding with a facet rhizotomy.

Indications and Rationale

Facet joint pain is most commonly related to degenerative spondylosis and arthropathy which presents as localized pain over the region of the degeneration [4]. A traumatic forced flexion or hyperextension can cause capsular stretch or joint compression can also cause injury to the facet joints [5, 6]. Facet joint pain typically presents as localized pain over the facet joint with myofascial radiating patterns that is worse with extension and rotation.

Along with clinical findings, diagnostic "paravertebral nerve blocks" (medial branch blocks or intra-articular facet blocks) are used to assist with the diagnosis of facet joint pain [4]. Local anesthetic is used to anesthetize the facet joint or the medial branch nerves that innervate the facet joints. If the blocks achieve 80 % or greater pain relief temporarily, then a patient is considered to be a good candidate for radiofrequency denervation of the medial branch nerves [7]. There is moderate evidence to support benefits of medial branch blocks. Randomized, placebo-controlled, and double-blinded studies have shown significant pain relief with radiofrequency nerve ablation, indicating strong evidence for its benefits [8]. Available evidence from randomized, controlled trials and observational studies for benefits of intra-articular facet joint injections is mixed and rated moderate to limited [9].

Techniques

Paravertebral Facet Blocks and Radiofrequency Ablations (Facet Rhizotomy)

The medial branch nerves are terminal divisions of the dorsal rami of each spinal nerve. They provide sensory sensation from the facet joints and motor innervation to the multifidi muscles. Each facet joint is innervated by the medial branch nerves at that vertebral level and the level above; thus it is important to block two sets of medial branch nerves for each facet joint.

In the cervical spine, the medial branch courses around the waist of the articular pillars. The patient can be placed in the prone or lateral decubitus position. The fluoroscopic beam is oriented with a slight tilt to line up the plane of the joint and the needle is guided towards the lateral aspect of the waist of the articular pillar. The fluoroscopic beam is then reoriented to a lateral position and the needle is advanced to the midpoint of the articular pillar (Figs. 12.1 and 12.2).

In the thoracic spine, the medial branches course over the superior aspect of the transverse process. Patients are placed in the prone position and the fluoroscopic beam is oriented in an AP or slightly oblique view. The needles are directed towards the superior aspect of the transverse process [10].

In the lumbar spine, the medial branch is at the junction between the superior articular process and the transverse process [11]. Patients are placed in the prone position and the fluoroscopic beam is oriented to square off the vertebral end plates in an AP or slightly oblique view. The spinal needles are directed towards the super-olateral aspect of the pedicle at the junction of the superior articular process and transverse processes (Figs. 12.3 and 12.4).

Fig. 12.1 AP fluoroscopic
view of right cervical
medial branch block

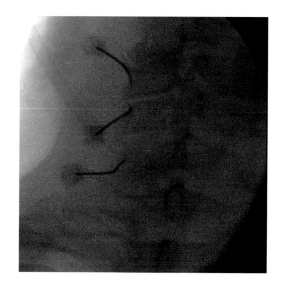

Fig. 12.2 Lateral
illustration of cervical
medial branch block. From
Fung DA et al. Injections
of the Cervical, Thoracic,
and Lumbar Spine. In:
Surgical Approaches to the
Spine, Watkins RG III and
Watkins RG, IV, eds.
Springer
New York;2015:389–409.
Reprinted with permission
from Springer

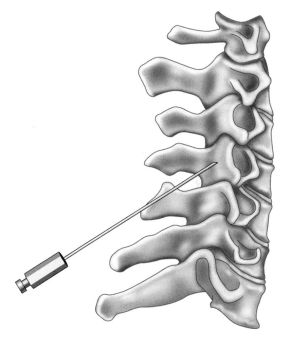

Radiofrequency ablation of the medial branches is performed at a similar location to the medial branch blocks. An insulated needle with an active tip is used to carry out the ablation. Sensory and/or motor stimulation are used to confirm placement of the needle near the medial branch nerves and away from the dorsal roots.

Fig. 12.3 AP fluoroscopic
view of left lumbar medial
branch block

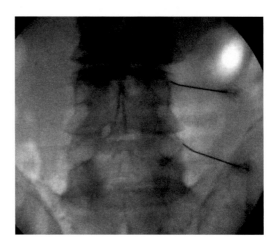

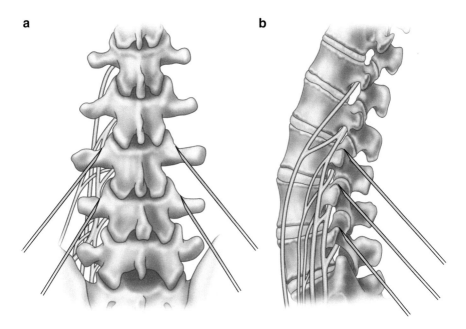

Fig. 12.4 AP and lateral medical illustration of bilateral lumbar medial branch block. From Fung
DA et al. Injections of the Cervical, Thoracic, and Lumbar Spine. In: Surgical Approaches to the
Spine, Watkins RG III and Watkins RG, IV, eds. Springer New York;2015:389–409. Reprinted
with permission from Springer

Fig. 12.5 AP fluoroscopic
view of bilateral lumbar
medial branch
radiofrequency ablation

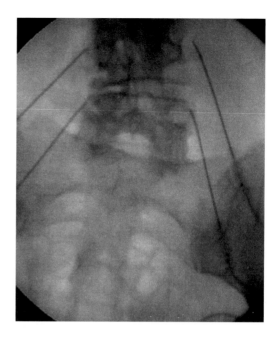

Local anesthetic is administered prior to the ablation and the ablation is typically
carried out at around 80 °C for a duration of 60–90 s [12] (Fig. 12.5).

Facet Joint Intra-Articular Injection

Cervical facet joint injections are performed with the patient lying prone and a
25–35 ° caudal tilt of the fluoroscopic beam to line up the facet joint space. The
needle is advanced towards and into the joint space, and slight resistance is felt
when the joint capsule is engaged. A lateral fluoroscopic view can be used to assess
the depth of the needle. Contract is used to confirm location of the needle tip in the
facet joint and 0.5–1 cc of medication is then typically injected to avoid distending
the joint capsule.

Thoracic facet joint injections are performed with the patient lying prone and the
fluoroscopic beam in a far (50–60 °) caudal tilt. Using fluoroscopic guidance the needle is directed towards the inferior articular process; once bone is contacted the needle
type is walked superiorly into the facet joint. Once needle is in place, contrast is used
to confirm the locations and approximately 1 cc of medication is typically injected.

Lumbar facet joint injections can be performed in two ways. Both require the
patient to be in a prone position. The traditional way is with the fluoroscopic beam
orientated obliquely approximately 20–30 ° to visualize the facet joint. The needle
is directed towards the facet joint and once entered contrast is injected to confirm
location and approximately 1–1.5 cc of medications is typically injected. The

author's preferred method is to keep the fluoroscopic beam in a direct AP position. The target is the posterior inferior aspect of the joint capsule. The needle is inserted in a medial to lateral, inferior to superior trajectory. The needle tip contacts the pars interarticularis of the inferior vertebrae, and then is marched up to the inferior aspect of the joint space. A step off can be appreciated when the joint is entered. This method is felt to be superior to the traditional intra-articular facet approach for safety and reproducibility. The tip is on bone throughout the procedure; therefore, the depth of the needle tip is known during the procedure, which makes it safe and easy to avoid spinal canal entry. The technique is reproducible from an anatomic perspective. The oblique fluoroscopic perspective of the lumbar facet joint can be deceiving. The joint line can often appear to be a flat line under fluoroscopy, but in reality, the joint is not a flat line, and can have scalloping traction osteophytes on the posterior lateral margin of the superior articular process blocking the access to the facet joint from the oblique approach.

Facet joint injections are relatively safe procedures in the right hands. Pain can temporarily worsen after injection due to muscle spasms, contact with the articular surface, or joint capsule expansion. Cervical injections can be risker due to the denser arrangement of nerves and arteries; nonparticulate steroids should be used to minimize the risk of arterial embolism. Another complication is injury to the spinal cord if the needle is placed too deeply and medially [8, 9].

Epidural Injections

The epidural space surrounds the dural sac and exiting spinal nerve roots within the spinal canal. The exiting spinal roots are typically the targets for epidural injections to treat radicular symptoms.

Indications and Rationale

A radicular referral pattern of pain caused by injury or irritation to a spinal nerve root is the primary indication for epidural injections. Radiculitis is often associated with dull aching centrally at the level of the exiting nerve root with sharp radiating pain along a dermatomal pattern that can be associated with numbness, paresthesia, and myotomal weakness. Proper history and physical exam should be correlated with imaging studies to visualize the pathology at the exiting nerve root. Electromyography (EMG) can also be used to confirm a diagnosis of radiculitis. Subjects with radiculitis and positive findings on EMG are reported to have improved functional outcomes from epidural steroid injections as compared to EMG-negative subjects [13]. Epidural steroid injections are accepted as a standard treatment for radiculitis and neurogenic claudication [14].

The American Society of Interventional Pain Physicians (ASIPP) guidelines advise that epidurals should be limited to a maximum of six per year and only repeated as medical necessary. Numerous studies have validated the efficacy and outcomes of caudal, interlaminar, and transforaminal steroid injections [15–18]. There is strong-to-moderate evidence supporting caudal and transforaminal epidural steroid injections [8]. Evidence for interlaminar injections is considered moderate to limited. However, multiple observational studies have shown positive results with all forms of epidural injections [8].

In order to meet CMS documentation requirements, providers must document moderate-to-severe pain, greater than 3/10, and functional impairment in activities of daily living. At least 4 weeks of failed conservative management must be adequately documented.

Accurate documentation of medication dosing, symptom location, as well as pre- and post-procedure response to the injection, including pain level and ability to perform previously painful movements, is also required [1].

Technique

Caudal, transforaminal, and interlaminar approaches to the epidural space are described.

Caudal Epidural Injection

The patient is placed in the prone position. The sacrum and sacral hiatus are identified using a lateral fluoroscopic view. A spinal or Tuohy epidural needle is advanced at a shallow angle in a cephalad direction into the sacral hiatus. A loss of resistance technique with a glass syringe and saline can be used to identify entrance of the needle through the sacral hiatus and into the epidural space. An epidural catheter can be advanced up to the desired level of injection or injectate can be administered into the lower caudal space with enough volume such that it spreads in a cephalad direction. Contrast solution is injected to confirm ideal placement in the epidural space without intravascular uptake and then the medications are injected. The needle should not be advanced past the S2 level to avoid the risk of dural puncture [19]. The risk of cauda equina syndrome is low, at around 2.7 per 100,000 epidural blocks [7].

Interlaminar Epidural Injection

The patient is placed in the prone position with slight flexion of the spine to help open up the intralaminar space (Fig. 12.6). AP fluoroscopy is used to visualize the intralaminar space and the lamina above and below. The spinal needle is advanced to just contact the superior aspect of the inferior lamina adjacent to the spinous process to confirm appropriate depth of the needle. The needle is then slowly walked off the lamina and advanced with a loss of resistance technique into the epidural

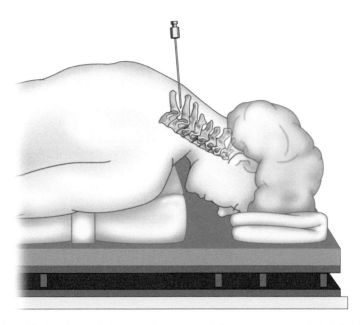

Fig. 12.6 Positioning for cervical interlaminal epidural injection. From Fung DA et al. Injections of the Cervical, Thoracic, and Lumbar Spine. In: Surgical Approaches to the Spine, Watkins RG III and Watkins RG, IV, eds. Springer New York;2015:389–409. Reprinted with permission from Springer

space (Fig. 12.7). Contrast is injection to confirm ideal placement of the needle and then medications are injected. The thoracic and cervical epidural space can be extremely narrow; thus entering at a more caudal interlaminar level and advancing an epidural catheter up to the desired level are often advised.

Aspiration is performed prior to injection of contrast to check for blood or CSF. The potential size of the dorsal epidural space is directly related to the volume of the spinal canal at the targeted level [20, 21] (Fig. 12.8).

Transforaminal Epidural Injection

The authors will present and prefer the retroneural method for transforaminal epidural steroid injections. The patient is placed in the prone position and an AP or oblique fluoroscopic view is used to direct the spinal needle from a lateral starting position medially towards the neural foramen. The needle is advanced obliquely toward the inferior lateral aspect of the pedicle at the junction of the transverse process and the pars. Lateral fluoroscopic imaging is then used to place the needle tip at the 10 o'clock position of the foramen, also known as the "safe triangle"

Fig. 12.7 Paramedian
approach for cervical
interlaminar epidural
injection. From Fung DA
et al. Injections of the
Cervical, Thoracic, and
Lumbar Spine. In: Surgical
Approaches to the Spine,
Watkins RG III and
Watkins RG, IV, eds.
Springer
New York;2015:389–409.
Reprinted with permission
from Springer

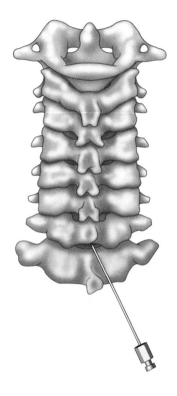

Fig. 12.8 AP fluoroscopic
view of cervical
interlaminar epidural
steroid injection with entry
point at the T1–T2
interlaminar space

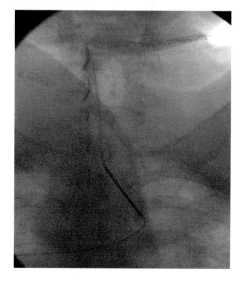

Fig. 12.9 AP fluoroscopic
view of lumbar
transforaminal epidural
steroid injection with
needles in place

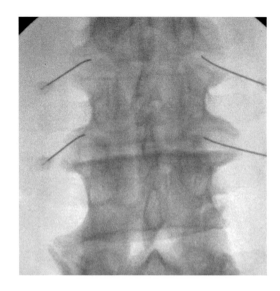

Fig. 12.10 Lateral
fluoroscopic view of
lumbar transforaminal
epidural steroid injection
with needles in place

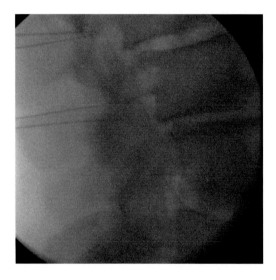

(Figs. 12.9, 12.10, 12.11, and 12.12). Cervical transforaminal epidural injections are not advised for unexperienced physicians; serious adverse events have been reported including paralysis, stroke, and death [22, 23].

Fig. 12.11 AP
fluoroscopic view of
lumbar transforaminal
epidural steroid injection
after administering contrast
and medications

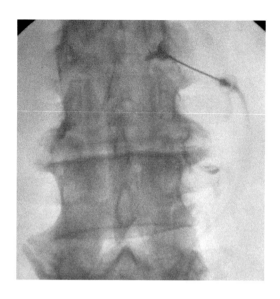

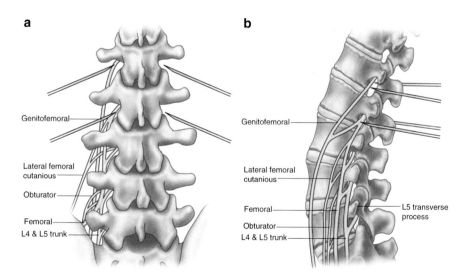

Fig. 12.12 AP and lateral medical illustration of lumbar transforaminal epidural steroid injection. From Fung DA et al. Injections of the Cervical, Thoracic, and Lumbar Spine. In: Surgical Approaches to the Spine, Watkins RG III and Watkins RG, IV, eds. Springer New York;2015:389–409. Reprinted with permission from Springer

Complications

Epidural injections are relatively safe procedures and complications are low. Previous studies have reported complications rates around 2.4 % with the most common complication being pain at the injection site [24]. Other studies have reported the incidence of a minor infection at 1–2 %, major infections 0.1–0.01 %, and the risk of epidural hematoma at less than 1 in 150,000 [25]. The risk of intravascular injection can be prevented by injecting contrast first to rule out intravascular placement but this is a possible complication and the use of nonparticulate steroid is recommended. A dural puncture can occur if the needle is advanced passing the epidural space; most patients will heal without intervention but if a dural leak persists it can be treated with staying supine, hydration, analgesics, and an autologous blood patch [26]. If the needle is advanced further into the dural space, contact with the spinal cord or nerve roots can occur. Epidural infections and epidural hematomas are rare occurrences that can lead to cauda equina syndrome. Extra care needs to be taken during left-sided injections between T8 and L1 because the artery of Adamkiewicz, the largest spinal segmental artery, lies at these levels in 60–80 % of patients [27, 28]. Certain steroid solutions now come with warning labels "not for epidural use." These are the same steroids that have been used in the epidural space for many years. The use of these products with this specific wording on the label in the epidural space is discouraged and very difficult to defend from a medical legal perspective.

Sacroiliac Joint Injections

The sacroiliac joint is a fibrocartilaginous joint formed by the connection between the sacrum and the ilium.

Indications

Sacroiliac (SI) joint pain typically presents as chronic axial low back pain that is localized to the lower back and buttock region. It is associated with leg length discrepancy, older age, inflammatory arthritis, scoliosis, previous spine surgery, pregnancy, and trauma. SI joint arthropathy is typically diagnosed on history and physical exam and with diagnostic SI joint injections.

In order to meet CMS documentation requirements, providers must document moderate-to-severe pain, greater than 3/10, and functional impairment in activities of daily living. At least 4 weeks of failed conservative management must be adequately documented. Accurate documentation of medication dosing, location, as well as pre- and post-procedure response to the injection, including pain level and ability to perform previously painful movement, is required. SI joint injections will be considered medically necessary when an injection is given with imaging confirmation for diagnostic or therapeutic purposes after conservative management has failed [1].

Evidence-Based Rationale

Physical exam and imaging findings are often nonspecific for the diagnosis of SI joint pain [29]. Many patients with SI joint pain have radiographically normal-appearing SI joints [30]. SI joint injections can serve as diagnostic and therapeutic injections [29, 31]. Clinical studies have demonstrated intermediate-term benefit for both intra- and extra-articular injection of steroid at the SI region [29].

Technique

The patient is placed in a prone position with a contralateral oblique fluoroscopic angulation. The needle is advanced from an inferior and medial entry point cephalad into the joint space. Contrast can be injected to confirm intra-articular placement, and then followed by the injectate. ASIPP guidelines recommend that joint injections be repeated only as necessary and limited to a maximum of six local anesthetic and steroid blocks per year [7]. If adequate relief of symptoms is obtained, then sacral lateral branch rhizotomy or fusion procedures can be performed for longer lasting relief.

Discography

Intervertebral discs consist of a central nucleus pulposus and a surrounding annulus fibrosis. Only the outer third of the disc has neural innervations and vascular supply. Degenerative disc disease or traumatic fissures in the annulus fibrosis are thought to lead to discogenic pain [7, 32].

Indications

Discogenic pain typically presents as axial low back pain at the level of the suspect disc. Discography is a diagnostic procedure used to diagnose discogenic pain or for preoperative planning to evaluate for internal disc disruption, recurrent herniations, and pseudoarthrosis and to determine spinal fusion levels [7]. Stimulation of intervertebral discs and the reproduction of patient's usual axial pain indicate a positive physiologic test for discogenic pain. A normal disc should not produce the patient's usual pain. Fluoroscopic evaluation of the contrast spread pattern or post-procedure CT or MRI can provide further radiologic evaluation of the internal anatomy of a disc [32].

Discography is considered medically necessary for evaluation of disc pathology in persons with persistent, severe low back pain and abnormal interspaces on MRI, where other diagnostic tests have failed to reveal clear confirmation of a suspected disc as the source of pain and surgical intervention is being considered. During the procedure, accurate documentation of volume of contrast injected, disc morphology, pressures, and concordant or discordant pain level is required [1].

Evidence-Based Rationale

Discography relies on the subjective provocation of patient's pain; due to this, clinical outcome data and peer-reviewed literature have published a wide range of results. Despite conflicting reports, discography does have applications in a number of clinical settings [7]. Cohen et al. published a comprehensive review of lumbar discography which reported discography to be the more accurate than other radiologic studies in detecting degenerative disc disease [32].

Technique

In lumbar discography the patient is placed in the prone position and a 25–35° oblique fluoroscopic angle is used to line up the superior articular process with the midline of the vertebral end plate. A two-needle technique is recommended using a 18-gauge needle followed by a 5–8 in. 22-gauge needle inserted through the 18-gauge needle to keep the needle tip as sterile as possible. The needle is advanced towards the superior articular process and walked just lateral off the superior articular process towards the midline of the disc. As the needle encounters the annulus there is increased resistance; at this point alternating AP and lateral fluoroscopy should be used to insure that the needle tip is advanced to the center of the disc. A mixture of radiographic contrast and antibiotics is then slowly injected to pressurize the disc and the patient is questioned regarding their symptoms. The morphologic features of the disc and contrast spread or leakage under fluoroscopy are also identified and recorded. Manometry can be used to monitor the opening pressure and the filling pressures. Discs that strongly reproduce the patients' typical pain at low-to-medium pressures are considered positive. Post-procedure CT or MRI imaging can be obtained within 2–3 h for further radiologic evaluation [33] (Figs. 12.13, 12.14, and 12.15).

Thoracic discography is similar in technique to lumbar discography but is only recommended for skilled proceduralists because of increased risk posed by the anatomy. In thoracic discography the needle is advanced into the disc through a hyperlucent region centered over the disc on oblique fluoroscopy. This hyperlucent region

Fig. 12.13 AP
fluoroscopic view of
lumbar discography

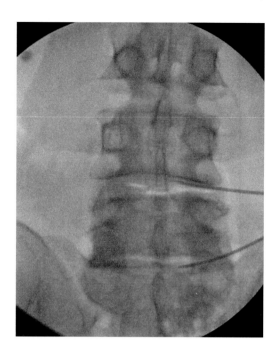

Fig. 12.14 Lateral
fluoroscopic view of
lumbar discography

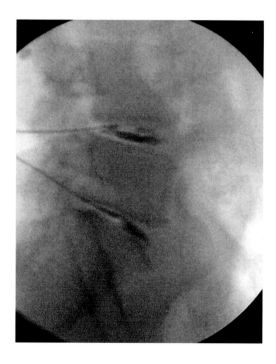

a   **b**

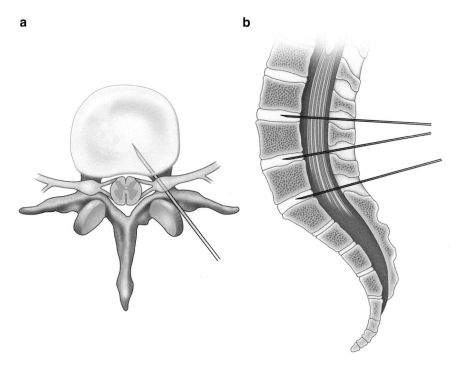

Fig. 12.15 Axial and lateral medical illustration of lumbar discography. From Fung DA et al. Injections of the Cervical, Thoracic, and Lumbar Spine. In: Surgical Approaches to the Spine, Watkins RG III and Watkins RG, IV, eds. Springer New York;2015:389–409. Reprinted with permission from Springer

is bordered by the superior and inferior vertebral endplates, laterally by the medial head of the rib and medially by the border of the pedicle.

Cervical discography is also only recommended for skilled proceduralists. The patient is placed in the supine position with the head slightly turned away from the needle entry point. A right-sided needle entry point is commonly used to avoid the esophagus. An oblique fluoroscopic view is used to visualize the uncinated process and neuroforamen. The needle should be directed towards the uncinated process. Once the uncinated process is contacted the needle is marched medially off the uncinated process into the disc. AP and lateral fluoroscopy should then be used to ensure proper placement into the midline of the disc (Figs. 12.16 and 12.17).

Complications

Although extremely rare, the most unique and serious complication of discography is discitis and it is difficult to treat with antibiotics due to the poor blood supply of the discs. Prophylactic IV antibiotics and antibiotics mixed in with contrast may

Fig. 12.16 AP
fluoroscopic view of
cervical discography

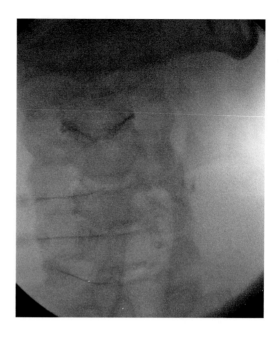

Fig. 12.17 Lateral
fluoroscopic view of
cervical discography

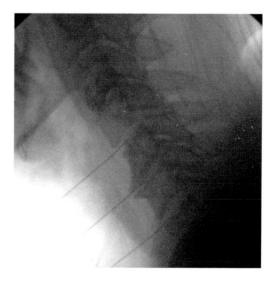

help decrease the risk of discitis [7, 34, 35]. Due to the subjective nature of discography, there can have a high false-positive rate [7, 34, 35]. "Control" or normal disc levels can be used to improve specificity of the study. However, Carragee et al. suggested that performing discography at a normal level may lead to accelerated progression of disc degeneration [36].

Minimally Invasive Interventional Procedures

Patients who have tried and failed conservative treatments and injections may be candidates for some of the more advanced minimally invasive interventional procedures. These procedures typically require small incisions and the implantation and administration of medical devices or biologic and synthetic materials. These procedures will be further discussed in future chapters but include and are not limited to spinal cord stimulation, peripheral nerve stimulation, intrathecal drug delivery, and vertebral augmentation for the treatment of advanced pain.

The Future of Interventional Procedures

The field of interventional pain management is constantly evolving with new minimally invasive procedures constantly being developed and adopted. The field of regenerative medicine is also emerging advocating biologic injections with stem cells and growth proteins. Further large-scale peer-reviewed studies on these subjects will be necessary to truly validate and confirm the safety and efficacy of such procedures.

References

1. CMS.gov Medicare Coverage Database. http://www.cms.gov/medicare-coverage-database/
2. Ay S, Evcik D, Tur BS. Comparison of injection methods in myofascial pain syndrome: a randomized controlled trial. Clin Rheumatol. 2010;29(1):19–23. Epub 2009 Oct 20.
3. Shankar H, Reddy S. Two- and three-dimensional ultrasound imaging to facilitate detection and targeting of taut bands in myofascial pain syndrome. Pain Med. 2012;13(7):971–5. doi:10.1111/j.1526-4637.2012.01411.x. Epub 2012 Jun 8.
4. Cohen SP, Raja SN. Pathogenesis, diagnosis, and treatment of lumbar zygapophysial (facet) joint pain. Anesthesiology. 2007;106(3):591–614.
5. Pearson AM, Ivancic PC, Ito S, Panjabi MM. Facet joint kinematics and injury mechanisms during simulated whiplash. Spine (Phila Pa 1976). 2004;29(4):390–7.
6. Cavanaugh JM, Ozaktay AC, Yamashita HT, King AI. Lumbar facet pain: biomechanics, neuroanatomy and neurophysiology. J Biomech. 1996;29(9):1117–29.
7. North RB, Han M, Zahurak M, et al. Radiofrequency lumbar facet denervation: analysis of prognostic factors. Pain. 1994;57:77–83.
8. Manchikanti L, Singh V, Kloth D, et al. Interventional techniques in the management of chronic pain: Part 2.0. Pain Physician. 2001;4(1):24–98.
9. Lynch MC, Taylor JF. Facet joint injection for low back pain. A clinical study. J Bone Joint Surg Br. 1986;68:138–41.
10. Bogduk N. International spinal injection society guidelines for the performance of spinal injection procedures. Part 1: Zygapophysial joint blocks. Clin J Pain. 1997;13(4):297–302.
11. Wallace MS, Moeller-Bertram T. Facet joint and epidural injections. Minimally invasive spine surgery. 2009: 99–104.

12. Niemistö L, Kalso E, Malmivaara A, Seitsalo S, Hurri H, Cochrane Collaboration Back Review Group. Radiofrequency denervation for neck and back pain: a systematic review within the framework of the Cochrane collaboration back review group. Spine (Phila Pa 1976). 2003;28(16):1877–88.
13. Annaswamy TM, Bierner SM, Chouteau W, Elliott AC. Needle electromyography predicts outcome after lumbar epidural steroid injection. Muscle Nerve. 2012;45(3):346–55.
14. Cohen SP, Bicket MC, Jamison D, Wilkinson I, Rathmell JP. Epidural steroids: a comprehensive, evidence-based review. Reg Anesth Pain Med. 2013;38(3):175–200. doi:10.1097/AAP.0b013e31828ea086.
15. Roberts ST, Willick SE, Rho ME, Rittenberg JD. Efficacy of lumbosacral transforaminal epidural steroid injections: a systematic review. PM R. 2009;1(7):657–68.
16. Abdi S, Datta S, Trescot AM, Schultz DM, Adlaka R, Atluri SL, Smith HS, Manchikanti L. Epidural steroids in the management of chronic spinal pain: a systematic review. Pain Physician. 2007;10:185–212.
17. Benny B, Azari P. The efficacy of lumbosacral transforaminal epidural steroid injections: a comprehensive literature review. J Back Musculoskelet Rehabil. 2011;24(2):67–76.
18. Macvicar J, King W, Landers MH, Bogduk N. The effectiveness of lumbar transforaminal injection of steroids: a comprehensive review with systematic analysis of the published data. Pain Med. 2013;14(1):14–28. doi:10.1111/j.1526-4637.2012.01508.x. Epub 2012 Oct 30.
19. Soleiman J, Demaerel P, Rocher S, Maes F, Marchal G. Magnetic resonance imaging study of the level of termination of the conus medullaris and the thecal sac: influence of age and gender. Spine (Phila Pa 1976). 2005;30(16):1875–80.
20. Cheng PA. The anatomical and clinical aspects of epidural anesthesia. Anesth Analg. 1963;42:398–406.
21. Husemeyer RP, White DC. Topography of the lumbar epidural space. A study in cadavers using injected polyester resin. Anaesthesia. 1980;35(1):7–11.
22. MacMahon PJ, Eustace SJ, Kavanagh EC. Injectable corticosteroid and local anesthetic preparations: a review for radiologists. Radiology. 2009;252(3):647–61. doi:10.1148/radiol.2523081929.
23. Scanlon GC, Moeller-Bertram T, Romanowsky SM, Wallace MS. Cervical transforaminal epidural steroid injections: more dangerous than we think? Spine (Phila Pa 1976). 2007; 32(11):1249–56.
24. McGrath JM, Schaefer MP, Malkamaki DM. Incidence and characteristics of complications from epidural steroid injections. Pain Med. 2011;12(5):726–31. doi:10.1111/j.1526-4637.2011.01077.x. Epub 2011 Mar 10.
25. Goodman BS, Posecion LWF, Mallempati S, Bayazitoglu M. Complications and pitfalls of lumbar interlaminar and transforaminal epidural injections. Curr Rev Musculoskelet Med. 2008;1:212–22.
26. Turnbull DK, Shepherd DB. Post-dural puncture headache: pathogenesis, prevention and treatment. Br J Anaesth. 2003;91(5):718–29.
27. Bley TA, Duffek CC, François CJ, Schiebler ML, Acher CW, Mell M, Grist TM, Reeder SB. Presurgical localization of the artery of Adamkiewicz with time-resolved 3.0-T MR angiography. Radiology. 2010;255(3):873–81. doi:10.1148/radiol.10091304.
28. Glaser SE, Shah RV. Root cause analysis of paraplegia following transforaminal epidural steroid injections: the 'unsafe' triangle. Pain Physician. 2010;13(3):237–44.
29. Foley BS, Buschbacher RM. Sacroiliac joint pain: anatomy, biomechanics, diagnosis, and treatment. Am J Phys Med Rehabil. 2006;85(12):997–1006.
30. Dreyfuss P, Dreyer SJ, Cole A, Mayo K. Sacroiliac joint pain. J Am Acad Orthop Surg. 2004;12(4):255–65.
31. Forst SL, Wheeler MT, Fortin JD, Vilensky JA. The sacroiliac joint: anatomy, physiology and clinical significance. Pain Physician. 2006;9(1):61–7.
32. Cohen SP, Larkin TM, Barna SA, Palmer WE, Hecht AC, Stojanovic MP. Lumbar discography; a comprehensive review of outcome studies, diagnostic accuracy and principles. Reg Anesth Pain Med. 2005;30(2):163–83.

33. Wolfer LR, Derby R, Lee JE, Lee SH. Systematic review of lumbar provocation discography in asymptomatic subjects with a meta-analysis of false-positive rates. Pain Physician. 2008;11:513–38.
34. Bogduk N, editor. International spine intervention society practice guidelines for spinal diagnostic and treatment procedures. 1st ed. San Francisco: International Spine Intervention Society; 2004. p. 20–46. ISBN 0-9744402-0-5.
35. Mathis JM, Golovac S. Image-guided spine interventions. 2nd ed. New York: Springer; 2010. p. 107–46. ISBN 9781441903525.
36. Carragee EJ, Don AS, Hurwitz EL, Cuellar JM, Carrino JA, Herzog R. Does discography cause accelerated progression of degeneration changes in the lumbar disc: a ten-year matched cohort study. Spine. 2009;34(21):2238–45.

Chapter 13
Neuromodulation

Kasra Amirdelfan

Key Points

- Neuromodulation is quickly evolving to keep pace with patients' needs.
- Advancements in neuromodulation include paresthesia-free therapies, novel neuraxial targets, innovative waveforms and frequencies and new intrathecal dosing regimens and pump platforms.
- Positioning of candidacy for advanced pain care therapies and placement in the pain care algorithm is evolving by moving away from salvage therapy, with earlier intervention improving treatment efficacy and safety.
- Intrathecal therapy is enjoying a rapidly evolving strategy and new offerings may provide improved accuracy.

Introduction

The efficient, effective, and long-term treatment of chronic pain has continued to be a challenging issue in modern medicine [1]. Until recently, the armamentarium of choices for treatment has been limited to rehabilitation, medications, injections, and nerve ablation. The developments in neuromodulation over the past four decades have been key in emerging this technology as one of the best-studied and most effective choices for the long-term control of chronic pain.

The North American Neuromodulation Society defines neuromodulation as a therapeutic alteration of activity, either through stimulation or medication, both of

K. Amirdelfan, M.D. (✉)
Medical Director & Director of Research,
IPM Medical Group, Inc., Walnut Creek, CA, USA

© Springer International Publishing Switzerland 2016
S.M. Falowski, J.E. Pope (eds.), *Integrating Pain Treatment into Your Spine Practice*, DOI 10.1007/978-3-319-27796-7_13

131

which are introduced by implanted devices [2]. Neuromodulation devices are not only used for the treatment of acute and chronic pain. Their utilization is also quite important in other conditions, such as epilepsy, spasticity, and movement disorders, including the emerging field of prosthetic neuromodulation [2].

Spinal cord stimulation (SCS) is arguably the best known and most utilized neuromodulation device for the treatment of chronic pain in the USA and around the world [3]. As such, it has also been extensively studied for both safety and efficacy. In 1967, Shealy and Mortimer were the first to describe the treatment of pain, via electrical stimulation, with electrodes placed directly over the dorsal column, in the intrathecal space of a patient with terminal cancer [4]. The first epidural placement of electrodes over the dorsal column was described in 1971. Shimogi and colleagues reported improved pain control with this type of placement [5]. Their efforts paved the way for the advances achieved in this field.

Over the next four decades, the spinal cord stimulator has undergone numerous iterations, including rechargeable internal power generators (IPGs), multiple contacts and electrodes, as well as improved software, in order to maximize their efficiency [6]. Throughout their evolution thus far, spinal cord stimulators have become increasingly effective in controlling neuropathic pain in the trunk and limbs. However there is now new evidence for sustained control of low back pain as well [7]. These devices are now an integral piece of the standard of care for long-term pain control in the USA and the rest of the developed world.

The first intrathecal delivery of drug has been credited to Leonard Corning, who administered intrathecal (IT) local anesthetic for pain control in 1885 [8]. The modern format of the intrathecal drug delivery systems (IDDS) began to gain traction after Wang and colleagues described improved pain control for cancer patients with IT morphine in 1979 [9]. The efficacy of IT opioid analgesic infusion has been verified in a number of published studies, as well as our own clinical practices. The best improvement with opioid IDDS is evident in chronic pain patients who have had analgesia, with conservative dosing of systemic opioid medications, but were intolerant to their side effects [10]. Alternatively, in patients with a suboptimal response to systemic or IT opioid medications, ziconotide has proven to be effective as a novel IT agent for pain control [11].

Evidence

Although both intrathecal drug delivery systems (IDDS) and spinal cord stimulators (SCS) are commonly utilized in the treatment of chronic pain, SCS has enjoyed a recent insurgence in technical advancements and popularity as the neuromodulation device of choice. This is based on its ease of implementation, efficacy, and low complication rates reported in the literature [12]. Nonetheless, IDDS continues to be a viable and strong choice for patients who would be candidates for neuromodulation. However, IDDS is typically reserved for patients who have either been inappropriate candidates for SCS, due to various relative or absolute contraindications, or failed an SCS trial [13].

Spinal Cord Stimulation

Since their inception, the SCS devices have been extensively studied for safety and efficacy [14]. SCS is commonly used in post-lumbar laminectomy syndrome (FBSS) patients, after surgical options have been exhausted and the patient continues to have low back and/or limb pain. However, there is evidence in the literature indicating that SCS may be a more effective and less costly modality than re-operation for patients with a history of previous lumbar surgery [15]. Moreover, patients who underwent an SCS implantation, after such re-operation, had a less optimal outcome with SCS [15]. SCS has also been shown to be extremely cost effective when compared with conventional medical management of FBSS patients, among many other diagnoses where SCS would be indicated [16].

Primary Indications for SCS
Failed back surgery syndrome (FBSS)
    Lumbar radiculopathy
    Arachnoiditis
    Complex regional pain syndrome (CRPS)
    Causalgia
    Cervical radiculopathy
    Diabetic and peripheral neuropathy

The low complication rates associated with these implants have been reported in multiple studies [12]. More importantly, the efficacy, in terms of optimal pain control [17], reduction in medications [14], and increase in function, including return to work [18], has also been demonstrated in the published literature.

SCS devices have enjoyed increasing popularity not only based on their long-term pain control, but also for their safety (Fig. 13.1). There is a significant lack of similar strong evidence for other treatment options, including opioids [1] and interventional management techniques, such as epidural injections [19]. Furthermore, there is research suggesting that earlier intervention with SCS after spinal surgery may be significantly more successful versus later consideration in the treatment algorithm [17].

The literature also suggests that SCS may be more effective than re-operation in patients who have undergone a technically successful spinal surgery [20]. As such, a growing number of pain physicians believe that SCS may not only be considered

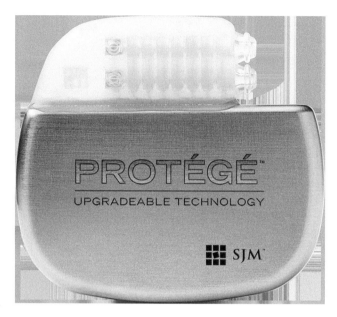

Fig. 13.1 Tonic SCS generator with software upgrade capability (courtesy of St. Jude Medical)

for patients with FBSS, but also for patients who have multilevel degenerative disc disease without a clear surgical option to alleviate their low back and leg pain.

Various SCS modalities currently available or under near-term investigation can be categorized as the following:

1. Tonic or traditional stimulation
2. Adaptive stimulation
3. High-frequency stimulation (HF-10 Therapy™)
4. Burst stimulation
5. Dorsal root ganglion stimulation (DRG)

Each of these categories of SCS contains unique properties and advantages as described below:

Tonic or Traditional Stimulation

Tonic SCS, also known as traditional stimulation or low frequency SCS, has been highly utilized around the world, as it was the pioneer modality in this category of neuromodulation. Tonic stimulation waveform frequency ranges between 1 and 50 Hz. It has been shown that tonic SCS is most effective within this range in the attenuation of the pain signal at the dorsal column [21]. Traditional stimulators depend on paresthesia mapping of the patient for a successful outcome. In other words, the paresthesia sensation will need to overlap the painful areas of the patient in order to attenuate their pain [22]. Therefore, intraoperative paresthesia mapping

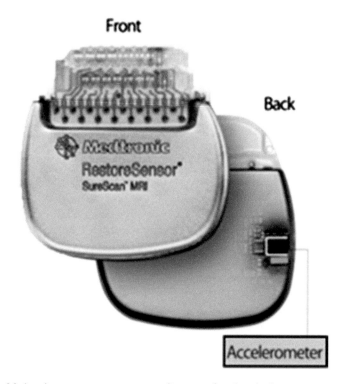

Fig. 13.2 Medtronic restore sensor generator. Courtesy of medtronic, Inc

for placement of the leads within the epidural space, based on Barolat mapping, is a requirement for this type of stimulation [22].

Adaptive Stimulation

Adaptive Stimulation was designed to address overstimulation and understimulation resulting from posture changes, thereby enhancing SCS therapy. Changes in body position cause the spinal cord to move within the intrathecal space resulting in variations in the distance between the spinal cord and stimulating electrodes [23]. The resulting change in distance between the spinal cord and the stimulating electrodes may cause transient overstimulation or understimulation which may require patient or clinician adjustment of stimulation parameters to accommodate changes in body position or physical activity [24].

The AdaptiveStim™ feature automatically adjusts the electrodes and stimulation parameters, including amplitude, in response to changes in body position or physical activity. These changes are detected by an integrated three-axis accelerometer and associated software contained in the neurostimulator (Fig. 13.2). Results from a multicenter, prospective randomized cross-over study show patient preference for

AdaptiveStim when compared to spinal cord stimulation without automatic adjustment [25]. With AdaptiveStim, 88.7% patients reported better pain relief and 90.1% reported better convenience compared to conventional stimulation.

High-Frequency Stimulation

A form of high-frequency SCS at 10,000 Hz (10 kHz), known as HF10™ therapy, has been the subject of growing interest with emerging published evidence in the literature. Van Buyten and colleagues first introduced the HF10 technology to pain physicians in a multicenter European study in 2013 [26]. They demonstrated significant improvement of back pain at 6 months, in this pilot study. Tiede and colleagues also reported similar results in the USA as part of an initial feasibility study [27].

A randomized, controlled trial (RCT) comparing HF10 stimulation to traditional (tonic) stimulation, the first of its kind in neuromodulation, was recently completed in the USA. This historic study demonstrated superior efficacy of HF10 therapy SCS over traditional (tonic-low frequency) SCS for both back and leg pain at 12 months. The results were presented at the 2014 North American Neuromodulation Society (NANS) meeting and the subsequently publsihed int he Journal of Anesthesiology [7]. There are no paresthesias perceived by the patient at 10,000 Hz. As such, HF10 therapy does not rely on paresthesia mapping for pain control. The advantages of this phenomenon, aside from its superiority for back and leg pain control, include eliminated negative positional effects of traditional SCS and loss of pain control due to loss of paresthesia overlap.

Burst Stimulation

The supporting theory for the efficacy of burst SCS is based on the inherent existence of neurons within the central nervous system (CNS) which produce action potentials in groups of "bursts." Such bursts, typically at a frequency of 500 Hz, are physiologically present in parallel to tonic action potentials in the CNS [28]. Studies have also demonstrated a more powerful response from burst than tonic stimulation, particularly in the activation of the cerebral cortex [29]. DeRidder and colleagues were able to demonstrate improved efficacy of burst SCS over traditional SCS for axial back pain [30]. Furthermore, burst stimulation does not produce paresthesias for the majority of its patients secondary to its sub-sensory amplitudes, which may achieve efficacy before the sensory thresholds are reached [31]. A randomized, placebo-controlled trial for failed back surgery syndrome patients published by Schu and colleagues established the efficacy of burst SCS vs. 500 Hz tonic SCS and placebo [31]. A multicenter US RCT of burst SCS vs. tonic stimulation is currently under way. Figure 13.3 depicts the various waveforms and frequencies for HF10, burst, and traditional stimulation.

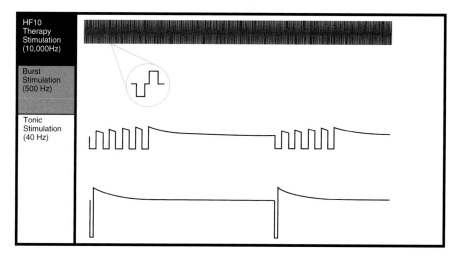

Fig. 13.3 SCS waveforms and frequencies

Fig. 13.4 DRG leads at the L5 level (courtesy of Kasra Amirdelfan, M.D.)

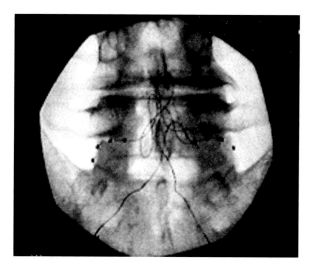

Dorsal Root Ganglion Stimulation (Fig. 13.4)

The dorsal root ganglion (DRG) has recently been established as a new target for SCS in the neuraxis, although it has been of interest as a target to treat chronic pain for some time [32]. The DRG is located bilaterally within the spine. The cell bodies for the primary afferent neurons are located directly caudal to the pedicles in the transforaminal space [33]. There are two main types of neurons (type A and B) within the DRG. The type B neurons are thought to be responsible for nociceptive sensation, whereas the type A neurons are largely responsible for touch, vibration, and proprioception [34].

The low amplitude of electrical stimulation at the DRG has been shown to promote growth factors involved in the regeneration of spinal neurons [35]. This promotion is mediated through specific growth factors, which are also associated with neuropathic pain. Electrical activity has been shown to modulate such growth factors [36]. As such, it is plausible that such neuro-secretory promotion via electrical stimulation may be responsible, in a direct or an indirect manner, for the attenuation of the pain signal at the DRG [37]. There is also evidence of wide dynamic range (WDR) neuron attenuation with DRG stimulation in the animal model, which could also be responsible for the analgesia with electrical stimulation at this structure [38].

In a single-arm, prospective pilot study, Deer and colleagues demonstrated up to 70 % pain relief in subjects suffering from chronic neuropathic pain with DRG spinal stimulation [39]. The long-term efficacy of the DRG SS has also been established in a number of studies. Liong and colleagues published the 12-month results of their multicenter European study, showing approximately 56 % overall pain relief in their subjects with intractable pain of the trunk and limbs [40]. A randomized RCT of DRG spinal stimulation versus tonic stimulation was recently completed in the USA. Finally, there is emerging evidence for the treatment of low back pain with DRG SCS placed at the L2 level [41]. Although promising, additional investigation is warranted for this utilization.

The study randomized patients in a 1:1 fashion with complex regional pain syndrome or peripheral causalgia of the lower extremity (defined as the iliac crest down), with a visual analog scale greater than 6, pain for at least 6 months, to treatment with either traditional SCS or DRG-SS, with endpoint of efficacy at 3 months and safety at 12 months.

152 patients were randomized, 146 were trialed (73 in each group). The results are compelling and demonstrated statistical superiority to SCS.

◦ 81.2 % of patients that underwent the trial with DRG experienced 50 % pain relief or greater at 3 months as compared to 55.7 % for SCS
◦ 74.2 % of the patients that underwent the trial with DRG experienced 50 % pain relief or greater at 12 months as compared to 53.0 % for SCS
◦ 93.3 % of patients that underwent the implant had 50 % pain relief or greater at 3 months, as compared to 72.2 % for SCS
◦ 86 % of the patients that underwent the implant had 50 % pain relief or greater at 12 months as compared to 70 % for SCS
◦ The DRG group demonstrated non-inferiority and superiority at 3 months when compared to SCS for all primary endpoints
◦ At 3 months, 70 % of the patients in the DRG group had at least 80 % pain reduction

These results are impactful, nearing the goal of a number needed to treat (NNT) of one. Moreover, there was no paresthesia difference noted with body position, as compared to signification differences with SCS, with precise stimulation (no bleed over paresthesia) in 94.5 % of patients. Subthreshold stimulation was very commonly achieved for DRG-SS. Migration rate is markedly lower for DRG-SS as compared to SCS as the stress-relief loop for the DRG system is placed within the epidural space, as compared to traditional SCS placement superficial to the lumbodorsal fascia.

Consider this: if a patient presents to clinic with CRPS or peripheral causalgia of the lower extremity, and you offer them a trial of DRG-SS, they have nearly a 75 % chance of getting at least 50 % relief at 12 months.

Intrathecal Drug Delivery System

The FDA has approved the intrathecal use of morphine and ziconotide for the treatment of moderate-to-severe pain. Ziconotide is a unique non-opioid calcium channel blocker with analgesic properties in the intrathecal space. The Polyanalgesic Consensus Committee (PACC), sponsored by INS, created a gold standard living document providing recommendations, as an evidence-based algorithm to introduce other medications as a solitary or combination therapy, for the treatment of both nociceptive and neuropathic pain [42]. The PACC recommendations not only include on-label uses of intrathecal agents; but they also include off-label medications as a single agent or in combination. At the time of this writing, the next iteration of the PACC is convening for projected publication in 2016.

Implementation

Spinal Cord Stimulation

The appropriate candidate for spinal cord stimulation is a patient who has not responded to conservative management. Moreover, such a patient does not have a viable surgical reparative option, which could potentially provide him/her with substantial long-term pain relief and increase in function. Medical and psychological comorbid factors will need to be taken into consideration for each patient. Once an SCS candidate has been identified, they are typically evaluated for absolute and relative medical contraindications for SCS [13]. Examples of such contraindications include, but are not limited to, uncontrolled diabetes, anticoagulation therapy, which cannot be safely interrupted, and spinal pathology preventing the safe implantation of the SCS device. The patient will then undergo a psychological evaluation to rule out any potential psychological contraindications, such as severe depression or secondary gain issues [43].

Once medically and psychologically cleared, the patient will typically undergo a percutaneous trial. The electrodes are placed, via percutaneous needles, at the target site within the epidural space. They are subsequently connected to an outside generator for the duration of the trial. The trial period may vary from 2 to 7 days, depending on the patient and physician preferences. Permanent trials, where the electrodes are subcutaneously implanted and connected to the outside generator via extensions, are more common in the European countries. The duration of such trials may last up to 30 days. There are advantages and disadvantages to each type of trial, which is beyond the scope of this chapter. However, length of trial past 5.9 days does not improve the rate of SCS conversion to the permanent therapy or permanent therapy outcomes [57]. Most physicians choose to perform the trials in the typical manner based on the standard of care in their geographical location, patient preference, and payer considerations.

During the trial, the patient will have the opportunity to fully evaluate his/her pain relief, along with any potential increase in function. The patient will then report the subjective and objective outcomes of the trial to the physician. During the trial, the representative for the SCS company commonly reprograms the patient for optimal stimulation as frequently as necessary. At the end of the trial, the patient will undergo an assessment regarding candidacy for the permanent therapy. The leads are typically "pulled" or removed in the office setting at the end of the trial visit.

One of the most medically appealing attributes of SCS therapy is the patient's option to undergo a percutaneous trial of the SCS system to establish its potential efficacy prior to a permanent implantation. The patients who choose not to proceed will either return to their established conventional regimen or be considered for other interventional treatment, such as IDDS.

Those who choose to undergo a permanent implantation will have the leads subcutaneously implanted, along with an internal power generator (IPG), under fluoroscopic guidance. The implanting physician may choose to implant the patient with percutaneous leads, which are available for all modalities described above, or place a paddle lead via laminotomy. Paddle leads are typically placed by a spine or neurosurgeon under direct visualization after a laminotomy near the target site in the spine. Paddle leads are currently only available for tonic and burst SCS, although others are actively developing paddles for their platforms as well. Paddle leads are thought to be more efficient due to the unidirectional nature of the electrodes [44] versus the percutaneous leads, which have cylindrical configurations delivering the electrical stimulation concentrically by 360°, although the risks and reversibility challenges are higher as compared to cylindrical percutaneous systems [58] (Figs. 13.5 and 13.6).

Another major advantage to SCS is the notion that the device implantation is reversible. The entire device may be explanted by the surgeon, should the patient choose to do so for any reason. The IPG and the electrodes can simply be removed from the subcutaneous pocket and the epidural space, respectively. The removal of a paddle lead may be more challenging. The scar formation around the paddles within the epidural space typically renders such implantations more complex for revisions or removals. Nonetheless, the procedure may be performed by an experienced spine or neurosurgeon in an expeditious manner, should the need present itself.

The most common complications reported in the literature with SCS implants are lead migration, infection, and lead fracture. Meaningful lead migration, defined as migration with loss of paresthesias or pain control, is by far the most common complication for SCS implants. The literature shows varying migration rates up to 22 % of the implanted leads [12]. However recent anchoring and surgical techniques

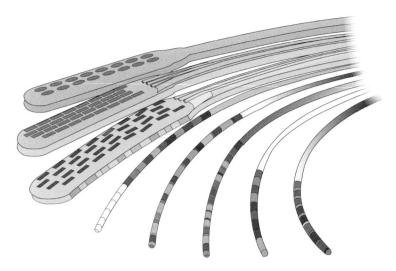

Fig. 13.5 SCS lead and paddle portfolio (courtesy of Boston Scientific Corporation)

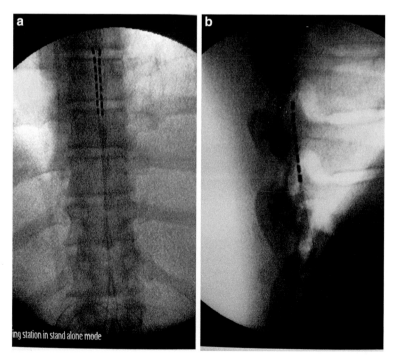

Fig. 13.6 Epidural placement of percutaneous traditional SCS leads (AP and lateral) (courtesy of Kasra Amirdelfan, M.D.)

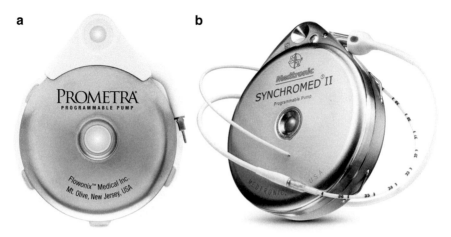

Fig. 13.7 A flowonix prometra pump (courtesy of Flowonix). b Medtronic synchromed II intrathecal pump catheter (reprinted with the permission of Medtronic, Inc. © 2013)

have mitigated lead migration to much lower rates. The rate of paddle versus percutaneous lead migration has been shown to be about the same [45]. However the paddle leads are reported to be more stable [46]. Infection rates for SCS are reported to be around 4–10 %, with some correlation to the patients' associated comorbidities, such as diabetes [47].

Intrathecal Drug Delivery System (Fig. 13.7)

Intrathecal drug delivery systems (IDDS) provide an alternative for medication delivery to the pain patient. Rauck and associates reported the best outcomes with IDDS for patients who were either refractory to oral or transdermal opioids or had intolerable side effects to such medications [10]. There is good evidence to support intrathecal delivery for both nociceptive and neuropathic pain from malignant and nonmalignant causes. These types of patients indeed form the majority of candidates for IDDS in a pain management practice. However, there are also specific pain diagnoses, which may respond better to IDDS, especially with combination therapy [48]. Currently, the patients who are commonly considered for IDDS for pain control can be divided into three specific categories:

1. Patients with intolerable side effects to systemic opioids with a favorable analgesic profile <120 morphine equivalents.
2. Patients who are refractory to systemic opioids with poor analgesic profile >120 morphine equivalents.
3. Patients who have failed spinal cord stimulation trials.

Once the physician has identified the appropriate patient, they typically undergo a psychological evaluation. Furthermore, the pros and cons of a permanent intrathecal pump implant and maintenance, as it pertains to the patient's specific analgesia and functional needs, are fully discussed. The patient will then undergo a trial of the intrathecal medication considered by the physician [42]. The trial may vary from a single shot of intrathecal injection or limited infusion to a more prolonged inpatient intrathecal infusion of the medication, up to 1 week. The mode of trial chosen depends on the physician's standard of practice and site of service requirements [49]. If optimal analgesia with a favorable side effect profile is achieved, the patient will undergo the device implantation, consisting of placement of the catheter and the reservoir. The catheter is placed intrathecally after it is typically inserted at the L2 or L3 level, below the conus medullaris, and directed over the dorsal columns around the T8 level for low back and leg pain targeting. The pump may be implanted subcutaneously in the lower quadrants of the abdomen, or elsewhere, depending on the patient and the physician's surgical preferences. The pump is filled periodically through the skin and the pump's central access port approximately every 2 to 3 months. The frequency of the refills depends on the dosing and concentration of the intrathecal regimen. Reprogramming occurs at the refills and intermittently as needed, based on the patient's specific requirements.

There are very few complications associated with the implantation procedure, especially in comparison to potential complications with systemic medication delivery [11]. One of the possible complications with IDDS therapy is a cerebrospinal headache after a catheter implantation or after a trial due to a cerebrospinal fluid leak. Fortunately, this complication is usually self-limited as the leak is gradually mitigated and halted by scar tissue around the catheter. The other common complications include infection, catheter dislodgment or migration, catheter fracture, and occlusion. The incidence of all such complications is reported to be less than 6 % [50]. Functional issues with the pump itself seldom occur; however, pocket infection and bleeding are reported as potential complications in and around the pump pocket.

A rare but serious complication of IDDS is the formation of a granuloma at the tip of the catheter. Such a granuloma is a noninfectious collection of cells that is hypothesized to result from an inflammatory response to the medication infusion at the distal end of the catheter within the intrathecal space. Catheter granulomas may compress the spinal cord, potentially constituting a compressive neurosurgical emergency [51]. Fortunately, the incidence of such granulomas is low and has been reported to be in the range of 0.1–5 %; however, such a wide range suggests that the actual incidence of granulomas is not well known [52]. As suggested, this may represent a pharmacokinetic failure instead of a pharmacodynamic challenge [59]. Along with continued improvements in catheter design and better understanding of the behavior of a foreign body and medications in the intrathecal space, the incidence of catheter inflammatory masses may be on the decline. Additional research is warranted to tabulate and understand the current incidence with newer technology.

Summary

Advanced neuromodulation devices for the treatment of chronic refractory pain have made great strides over the recent past. Neurostimulation, in particular, has enjoyed significant technological achievements over the past decade, with the emergence of more efficacious and specific therapies [27, 30, 40, 53]. This is especially true in the treatment of low back pain on a long-term basis, which has traditionally been extremely challenging to accomplish. HF10 therapy has already proven to be superiorly effective for the treatment of low back and leg pain, based on European and North American evidence with up to 2-year follow-up, so far [7, 53]. Emerging technologies such as dorsal root ganglion and burst stimulation have also rekindled hope for a more efficient treatment of chronic axial and limb pain. The results of their prospective US RCT studies are highly anticipated by both patients and experts in this field.

Intrathecal therapy has remained a cornerstone of chronic management of both malignant and nonmalignant pain. Advancing endeavors such as improved patient selection, pump and catheter design, new medications, and new dosing strategies will continue to provide an important tool for patients suffering from refractory pain [54].

Neuromodulation has already established its place in the realm of the standard of care for the treatment of chronic pain as a safe and effective step in the treatment algorithm. There is strong evidence suggesting that earlier intervention with neuromodulatory devices may improve outcomes and be more cost effective [16, 55, 56]. This type of modality has evolved to provide superior efficacy over a relatively short period of time. Neuromodulation and its exciting emerging technologies have created new horizons in the treatment goals of those physicians who care for patients with neuraxial pain. With increased efficacy, such modalities may eventually replace surgical repair of the spine for more complex patients with guarded prognoses regarding pain control and functional outcome. Improved efficacy, robust supportive research, as well as concomitant reduction of short- and long-term medical costs as compared with surgical intervention or conventional management will serve as the primary catalysts in the rapid adoption of neuromodulation in more surgical practices in the near future.

References

1. International Neuromodulation Society. [Online]. [cited 2015]. Available from: www.neuromodulation.com.
2. Kissin I. Long-term opioid treatment of chronic nonmalignant pain: unproven efficacy and neglected safety. J Pain Res. 2013;6:513–29.
3. Millennium Research Group. Neurostimulation Devices-U.S.-2014-Market Analysis. Executive Summary; 2014.
4. Shealy CN, Mortimer JT, Becker DP. Electrical inhibition of pain by stimulation of the dorsal columns: preliminary clinical report. Anesth Analg. 1967;46(4):489–91.

5. Shimoji K, Higashi H, Kano T, Asai S, Miroka T. Electrical management of intractable pain. Masui. 1971;20:444–7.
6. Dilorenzo DJ, Bronzino JD. Neuroengineering. Boca Raton: CRC Press; 2008.
7. Kapural L, Yu C, Doust M, Gliner B, Vallejo R, Sitzman T, Amirdelfan K, et al. Novel 10-kHz high-frequency therapy is superior to traditional low-frequency spinal cord stimulation for the treatment of chronic back and leg pain (The Senza Randomized Control Trial). Anesthesiology. 2015;3:4.
8. Deer T. Atlas of implantable therapies for pain management. New York: Springer; 2011.
9. Wang JK, Nauss LA, Thomas JE. Pain relief by intrathecally applied morphine in man. Anesthesiology. 1979;50:140–51.
10. Rauck R, Cherry D, Boyer M, Kosek P, Dunn J, Alo K. Long-term intrathecal opioid therapy with a patient-activated implanted delivery system for the treatment of refractory cancer pain. J Pain. 2003;4(8):441–7.
11. Smith H, Deer T. Safety and efficacy of intrathecal ziconotide in the management of severe chronic pain. Ther Clin Risk Manag. 2009;5:521–34.
12. Mekhail N, Matthews M, Nageeb F, Guiguis M, Mekhail M, Cheng J. Retrospective review of 707 cases of spinal cord stimulation: indications and complications. Pain Pract. 2011;11(2):148–53.
13. Neuromodulation Foundation. [Online]. [cited 2015]. Available from: www.neuromodfound. org.
14. Cameron T. Safety and efficacy of spinal cord stimulation for the treatment of chronic pain: a 20 year literature review. J Neurosurg. 2004;100(3):254–67.
15. North RB, Kidd D, Shipley J, Taylor RS. Spinal cord stimulation versus reoperation for failed back surgery syndrome: a cost effective and cost utility analysis based on a randomized, controlled trial. Neurosurgery. 2007;61(2):361–8.
16. Kumar K, Rizvi S. Cost-effectiveness of spinal cord stimulation therapy in management of chronic pain. Pain Med. 2013;14(11):1631–49.
17. Kumar K, Hunter G, Demeria D. Spinal cord stimulation in the treatment of chronic benign pain: challenges in treatment planning and present status, a 22-year experience. Neurosurgery. 2006;58:481–96.
18. Van Buyten JP, Van Zundert J, Vueghs P, Vanduffel L. Efficacy of spinal cord stimulation: 10 year experience in a pain center in Belgium. Eur J Pain. 2001;5:299–307.
19. Abdi S, Datta S, Trescot AM, Schultz DM, Adlaka R, Atluri SL, et al. Epidural steroids in the management of chronic spinal pain: a systematic review. Pain Physician. 2007;10(1):185–212.
20. North R, Kidd DH, Farrokhi F, Piantadosi SA. Spinal cord stimulation versus repeated lumbosacral spine surgery for chronic pain: a randomized controlled trial. Neurosurgery. 2005;56:98–106.
21. Schecter R, Yang F, Xu Q, Cheong YK, He SQ, Srdulla A, et al. Conventional and kilohertz-frequency spinal cord stimulation produces intensity- and frequency-dependent inhibition of mechanical hypersensitivity in a rat model of neuropathic pain. Anesthesiology. 2013;119(2): 422–32.
22. Barolat G, Massaro F, He J, Zeme S, Ketcik B. Mapping of sensory responses to epidural stimulation of the intraspinal neural structures in man. J Neurosurg. 1993;78(2):233–9.
23. Holsheimer J, den Boer JA, Struijk JJ, Rozeboom AR, 1994. MR assessment of the normal position of the spinal cord in the spinal canal. AJNR 15(5), 951–9.
24. Ross E, Abejon D. Improving patient experience with spinal cord stimulation: implications of position-related changes in neurostimulation. Neuromodulation. 2014;17 Suppl 1:36–41.
25. Schultz DM, Webster LR, Kosek P, Dar U, Tan Y, Sun M. Sensor-driven position-adaptive spinal cord stimulation for chronic pain. Pain Physician. 2012;15(1):1–12.
26. Van Buyten JP, Al-Kaisy A, Smet I, Palmisani S, Smith T. High frequency spinal cord stimulation for the treatment of chronic back pain patients: results of a multicenter European clinical study. Neuromodulation. 2013;16(1):59–65.
27. Tiede J, Brown L, Gennady G, Vallejo R, Yearwood T, Morgan D. Novel spinal cord stimulation parameters in patients with predominant back pain. Neuromodulation. 2013;16:370–5.

28. Oswald AM, Chacron M, Dorian B, Bastian J, Maler L. Parallel processing of sensory input by burst and isolated spikes. J Neurosci. 2004;24(18):4351–62.
29. Shemn SM. Tonic and burst firing: dual modes of thalamocortical relay. Trends Neurosci. 2001;24(2):122–6.
30. DeRidder D, Vanneste S, Plazier M, van der Loo E, Menovsky T. Burst spinal cord stimulation: towards paresthesia free pain suppression. Neurosurgery. 2010;66(5):986–90.
31. Schu S, Slotty P, Bara G, Von Knopp M, Edgar D, Veper J. Effectiveness of burst spinal cord stimulation patterns for the treatment of failed back surgery syndrome. Neuromodulation. 2014;17:443–50.
32. Pope JE, Deer TR, Kramer J. A systematic review: current and future directions of dorsal root ganglion therapeutics to treat chronic pain. Pain Med. 2013;14(10):1477–96.
33. Deer T, Krames ES, Mekhail N, et al. The appropriate use of neurostimulation: new and evolving neurostimulation therapies and applicable treatment for chronic pain and selected disease states. Neuromodulation. 2014;17:599–615.
34. Kishi M, Tannabe K, Schmelzer JD, Low PA. Morphometry of dorsal root ganglion in chronic experimental diabetic neuropathy. Diabetes. 2002;51:819–24.
35. SISKEN BF, Walker J, Orgel M. Prospects of clinical applications of electrical stimulation for nerve regeneration. J Cell Biochem. 1993;51:404–9.
36. Aaron RK, Boyan BD, Ciombor DM, Schwartz Z, Simon BJ. Stimulation of growth factors by electric or electromagnetic fields. Clin Orthop Relat Res. 2004;429:30–7.
37. Krames ES. The dorsal root ganglion in chronic pain and as a target for neuromodulation. Neuromodulation. 2015;18:24–32.
38. Fei Y, Chen Z, Qian X, Vinod T, Shao-Qiu H, Yun W, et al. Electrical stimulation of the dorsal root entry zone attenuates wide dynamic range neuronal activity in rats. Neuromodulation. 2015;18(1):33–40.
39. Deer T, Grigsby E, Weiner R, Wilcosky B, Kramer J. A prospective study of dorsal root ganglion stimulation for the relief of chronic pain. Neuromodulation. 2013;16(1):67–72.
40. Liong L, Russo M, Frank H, Van Buyten JP, Smet I, Verrills P, et al. One year outcomes of spinal cord stimulation of the dorsal root ganglion in the treatment of chronic neuropathic pain. Neuromodulation. 2015;18(1):41–9.
41. Hugyen H. Prospective results of L2 dorsal root ganglion stimulation for the treatment of chronic low back pain in failed back surgery syndrome. In Oral Abstract at 2014 North American Neuromodulation Society Meeting, Las Vegas.
42. Deer T, Prager J, Levy R, Rathmel J, Burton A, Caraway D. Polyanalgesic consensus conference 2012: recommendations for the management of pain by intrathecal (intraspinal) drug delivery: report of an interdisciplinary expert panel. Neuromodulation. 2012;15:436–66.
43. Campbell C, Jamison R, Edwards R. Psychological screening/phenotyping as predictors for spinal cord stimulation. Curr Pain Heahache Rep. 2012;17(1):307.
44. Sears NC, Machado AG, Nagel SJ, Deogonkar M, Stanton-Hicks M, Rezai AR. Long-term outcomes of spinal cord stimulation with paddle leads in the treatment of complex regional pain syndrome and failed back surgery syndrome. Neuromodulation. 2011;14:312–8.
45. Kim DD, Vakharyia R, Kroll HR, Shuster A. Rates of lead migration and stimulation loss in spinal cord stimulation: a retrospective comparison of laminotomy versus percutaneous implantation. Pain Physician. 2011;14(6):513–24.
46. Pahapill P. Incidence of revision surgery in a large cohort of patients with thoracic surgical three column paddle leads: a retrospective case review. Neuromodulation. 2014.
47. Follett KA, Brootz-Marx RL, Drake JM, Dupen S, Schnieder SJ, Turner MS, et al. Prevention and management of intrathecal drug delivery and spinal cord stimulation system infections. Anesthesiology. 2004;100(6):1582–94.
48. Koulousakis A, Kuchta J, Bayarassou A, Sturm V. Intrathecal opioids for intractable pain syndromes. Acta Neurochir Suppl. 2007;97(1):43–8.
49. Dominguez E, Sahinler B, Bassam D. Predictive value of intrathecal narcotic trials for long-term therapy with implantable drug administration systems in chronic non-cancer pain patients. Pain Pract. 2002;2(4):315–25.

50. Knight K, Brand F, Mchaourab A, Veneziano G. Implantable intrathecal pumps for chronic pain: highlights and updates. Croat Med J. 2007;48(1):22–34.
51. Arnold P, Harsh V, Oliphant S. Spinal cord compression secondary to intrathecal catheter-induced granuloma: a report of 4 cases. Evid Based Spine Care J. 2011;2(1):57–62.
52. Deer T. A retrospective analysis of intrathecal granuloma in chronic pain patients: a review of the literature and report of a surveillance study. Pain Physician. 2004;7:225–8.
53. Al-Kaisy A, Van Buyten JP, Smet I, Palmisani S, Pang D. Sustained efficacy of 10 kHz high frequency stimulation for patients with chronic low back pain: 24 month results of a prospective multicenter study. Pain Med. 2014;15(3):347–54.
54. Grider J, Harned M, Etscheitd M. Patient selection and outcomes using a low-dose intrathecal trialing method for chronic non-malignant pain. Pain Physician. 2011;14:343–51.
55. Kumar K, Hunter G, Demeria DD. Treatment of chronic pain by using intrathecal drug therapy compared with conventional pain therapies: a cost effectiveness analysis. J Neurosurg. 2002;97(4):803–10.
56. Poree L, Krames ES, Pope J, Deer TR, Levy R, Schultz L. Spinal cord stimulation as treatment for complex regional pain syndrome should be considered earlier then last resort therapy. Neuromodulation. 2013;16(2):125–41.
57. Chincholkar M, Eldabe S, Strachan R. Prospective analysis of the trial period for spinal cord stimulation treatment for chronic pain. Neuromodulation. 2011;14(6):523–8. discussion 528–9.
58. Levy R, Henderson J, Slavin K. Incidence and avoidance of neurologic complications with paddle type spinal cord stimulation leads. Neuromodulation. 2011;14(5):412–22. discussion 422.
59. Pope JE, Deer TR. Intrathecal pharmacology update: novel dosing strategy for intrathecal monotherapy ziconotide on efficacy and sustainability. Neuromodulation. 2015. doi:10.1111/ner.12274.

Chapter 14
Intrathecal Therapy for Chronic Spine Pain

Melinda M. Lawrence and Salim M. Hayek

Key Points

- IT therapy is not considered first-line therapy and should be considered once more conservative measures for intractable spine pain have failed or are not tolerated.
- Appropriate patient selection is critical for successful outcomes with IT therapy.
- IDDSs have proven to be beneficial in the treatment of chronic spine pain. FBSS and VCFs are the most common indications for IDDSs in chronic spine pain patients.
- The two drugs approved by the FDA to treat chronic pain in the IT space are morphine and ziconotide. Commonly used IT medications for the treatment of chronic pain include other opioids (hydromorphone, fentanyl); bupivacaine, a local anesthetic; and clonidine, an alpha 2 adrenergic agonist.
- When utilizing an IDDS it is important to have in-depth knowledge of the neuraxial space, CSF flow dynamics, indications, IT medications, device matters, and potential complications.

Patient Selection

An IDDS is an invasive and costly treatment option and therefore is not first-line therapy. A stepwise approach should be taken when considering a patient for an IDDS. Patients considered for an IDDS should first undergo more conservative

M.M. Lawrence, M.D. (✉) • S.M. Hayek, M.D., Ph.D.
Department of Anesthesiology, Division of Pain Medicine, Case Western Reserve University,
University Hospitals Case Medical Center, 11100 Euclid Ave., Cleveland, OH 44106, USA
e-mail: Melinda.Lawrence@UHhospitals.org; salim.hayek@uhhospitals.org

© Springer International Publishing Switzerland 2016   149
S.M. Falowski, J.E. Pope (eds.), *Integrating Pain Treatment into Your Spine
Practice*, DOI 10.1007/978-3-319-27796-7_14

treatment options which may include physical therapy, rehabilitation, pharmaco-therapy (over-the-counter medications, adjuvant pain medications, oral and trans-dermal opioids), cognitive and behavioral therapy, as well as alternative therapies. When selecting a patient for IT therapy one should consider a patient who has failed more conservative treatment options, is unable to tolerate pain medications due to side effects or is unable to obtain adequate relief with oral or transdermal medica-tions, has spinal anatomy that allows for placement of an IT catheter, is medically stable without untreated infectious processes or bleeding disorders, is mentally stable without untreated depression or anxiety disorders, and do not suffer from significant personality disorders [1]. Patients should undergo a psychological evalu-ation and a trial of IT therapy prior to permanent implant of an IDDS [2]. Another important factor when considering IT drug delivery is age, especially in chronic noncancer pain. Over time patients develop an increasing tolerance to IT opioids which requires further dose escalation. The issue of tolerance and dose escalation with IDDSs is an issue especially in younger patients [3]. Dose escalation is less of an issue in those patients older than 50 [3].

Indications

The Food and Drug Administration (FDA) approves the use of IDDSs in patients with moderate-to-severe pain due to cancer and noncancer causes. In those who suf-fer from noncancer causes the most common origin of pain is the spine. Common indications for chronic noncancer pain are post-laminectomy syndrome, failed back surgery syndrome (FBSS), vertebral compression fractures (VCF), spinal stenosis, spondylosis, and spondylolisthesis. Other indications for IDDSs are complex regional pain syndrome, neuropathy, rheumatoid arthritis, chronic abdominal pain (chronic pancreatitis), chest wall pain, and cancer pain [4–14].

Cerebrospinal Fluid Dynamics

An IDDS delivers medication to the cerebrospinal fluid (CSF) in the IT space where it is then distributed and ultimately diffuses to the site of action. Several factors play a role in the distribution of IT drug which include CSF flow, drug dose, drug vol-ume, rate of administration, and drug solubility. Flow-sensitive imaging techniques such as a phase-contrast MRI have allowed for qualitative and quantitative assess-ment of CSF flow [15]. Advanced imaging has revealed that the majority of CSF movement is due to pulsatile flow rather than bulk flow as previously thought [16–18]. The pulsatile flow of CSF in the spinal column is mainly due to arterial pulsa-tions and changes in intrathoracic pressure with respiration [15, 19–21]. There is cranial CSF flow in diastole and caudad flow during systole in the cervical and cervicothoracic regions; the direction of the CSF flow is a result of the arterial pulsations. In the lower thoracic spine respiratory influence is the predominant factor affecting flow [4, 19, 22]. During deep inspiration CSF moves cephalad while exhalation moves CSF caudad [23]. Medications delivered via IDDS are of low volume and slowly infused (typically <0.5 mL/day), which along with CSF flow dynamics limits the drug spread to just beyond the catheter tip [24, 25]. Variable anatomy that can occur in patients with spinal pain can further disrupt the pulsatile flow. However, ambulation or lack thereof may have differential effects on CSF flow and IT drug distribution [26].

Among medication factors including drug dose, drug volume, and rate of administration, lipid solubility may be the most important. Once the medication is delivered into the CSF via the IT catheter, it then diffuses through the pia arachnoid mater prior to diffusing into the target sites in lamina II of the dorsal horn (substantia gelatinosa; grey matter). A hydrophilic drug is more likely to penetrate into the cord and spread in the CSF, while a hydrophobic drug, which has a much larger volume of distribution, is more likely to be cleared from the IT space by diffusing into epidural fat and ultimately cleared by small vessels. Rate of administration and drug volume contribute to drug distribution and are derived primarily from literature on spinal anesthesia and cannot be directly applied to the long-term drug delivery with IDDSs (slow flow, low volume) [27]. Overall, CSF dynamics and the effect on IT drug are very complex and further exploration is needed.

Intrathecal Medications

There are three medications approved by the FDA for continuous use in the IT space, two medications are approved for the treatment of chronic pain, and one medication for the treatment of spasticity. The two medications approved to treat chronic pain in the IT space are morphine (Infumorph) and ziconotide (Prialt). Baclofen (Gablofen and Lioresal) is approved for IT use in the treatment of spasticity. Despite the fact that there are only two medications approved for continuous IT administration for chronic pain, there are other medications used for chronic pain that are considered to be standard of care. Commonly used IT medications for the treatment of chronic pain include other opioids (fentanyl, hydromorphone); bupivacaine, a local anesthetic; and clonidine, an alpha 2 adrenergic agonist. For the purpose of this chapter we focus on the medications used for the treatment of chronic noncancer pain, specifically spinal pain.

Throughout the chapter we discuss the PACC (Polyanalgesic Consensus Conference) guidelines in regard to IT medication recommendations. These guidelines can be used as a framework for interventional pain clinicians but they do have limitations and may not be applicable to every patient. The PACC guidelines were created through consensus by experts on IT therapy to help clinicians use IT therapy in a safe and effective way. One must also keep in mind that consensus guidelines and expert opinions represent the lowest level of evidence.

Opioids (Fentanyl, Hydromorphone, Morphine)

Opioids, when administered neuraxially, have a primary site of action on the opioid receptors in lamina II (substantia gelatinosa) in the dorsal horn of the spinal cord [28]. IT therapy is often considered for patients who cannot tolerate opioids due to adverse effects or have failed more conservative therapy [29]. An advantage of delivering opioids intrathecally is that there is a 60–300-fold decrease in dose required when converting from oral to IT [29]. Although the conversion rate for oral to IT is generally thought to be 300:1, there have been reports of conversion rates as low as 12:1 [30]. Conversion to IT administration can reduce or eliminate some of the systemic adverse effects associated with opioids and bypass the first-pass hepatic effect [29].

Although all IT opioids have the same site of action, the bioavailability is variable and primarily determined by the lipid solubility of each individual opioid drug [31]. Greater bioavailability in the dorsal horn is seen with hydrophilic drugs (hydromorphone and morphine) and less bioavailability with hydrophobic drugs (fentanyl). The greater bioavailability is due to the fact that hydrophilic drugs do not diffuse out of the CSF as readily, have a smaller volume of distribution, and are thus able to penetrate further into the grey matter. Hydrophobic opioids, on the other hand, diffuse more readily out of the CSF into the plasma where they are metabolized by the liver. Finally, opioid metabolites are eliminated from the system via renal excretion.

Opioids are indicated for the treatment of neuropathic and nociceptive pain according to the 2012 PACC guidelines [32]. Morphine is considered to be first-line therapy for neuropathic pain, while hydromorphone is second line, and fentanyl is third line. For nociceptive pain, morphine, hydromorphone, and fentanyl are all considered to be first-line therapy. It must be noted that these recommendations are likely based on consensus rather than evidence. Recommendations for IT opioid dosing are listed in the guidelines for bolus trialing, daily starting doses, and maximum daily dosing. Recommended starting doses for morphine, hydromorphone, and fentanyl are 0.1–0.5 mg/day, 0.02–0.5 mg/day, and 25–75 mcg/day, respectively. Maximum daily dosing recommended are 15 mg, 10 mg, and no known upper limit for morphine, hydromorphone, and fentanyl, respectively [32] (Table 14.1).

In contrast to the traditional method of using IT therapy in highly opioid tolerant patients, there is more novel concept of "microdosing" or using "low-dose" IT opioids. Microdosing involves weaning down opioid medication prior to the trial and

Table 14.1 Adapted from PACC 2012 recommendations for IT opioid dosing [32]

	Starting dose	Maximum daily dose	Maximum concentration ()
Morphine	0.1–0.5 mg/day	15 mg	20 mg/mL
Hydromorphone	0.02–0.5 mg/day	10 mg	15 mg/mL
Fentanyl	25–75 mcg/day	No known upper limit	10 mg/mL

implant to minimize the initial IT opioid dose. Two studies with lower initial IT opioid dosing reported sustained pain relief and limited IT dose escalation [22, 33]. Microdosing IT opioids is an attractive concept because it can decrease the potential adverse effects associated with high-dose IT opioids. Although there is some evidence to support microdosing, further research including prospective randomized control trials is needed.

Drug-related adverse effects for opioids include respiratory depression, peripheral edema, hormonal changes, tolerance, opioid-induced hyperalgesia, constipation, pruritus, and granuloma formation [34].

A granuloma is a sterile inflammatory mass found at the tip of an IT catheter. Granuloma formation has been associated with the use of high-dose opioids in the intrathecal space. Granuloma formation is most commonly associated with high-dose morphine but has also been reported with hydromorphone [35]. A granuloma may be suspected if IT therapy is no longer working or less effective despite dose escalation, there is new onset of intractable pain, and in the setting of new neurologic symptoms. If a granuloma is suspected an MRI with and without contrast should be ordered to evaluate. Treatment consists of removing the IT medication and refilling the pump with normal saline, usually for 6 months [35]. Beagle dog experiments show evidence of granuloma regression and near resolution with intrathecal infusion of preservative-free normal saline [36]. To minimize the chance of developing a granuloma one should use the lowest effective dose of opioid and the lowest concentration of opioid [35]. The utilization of nonopioid adjuvants, particularly bupivacaine, may help in limiting IT opioid dose escalation [37]. Granulomas are known to recur in patients who are re-exposed to granuloma-inducing opioids [38]. Fentanyl has not been associated with granuloma formation and may be a useful option in properly selected patients.

Ziconotide

Ziconotide is a synthetic version of a 25 amino acid polybasic peptide found in the venom of a marine snail (*Conus magus*) that selectively blocks the presynaptic N-type Ca^{2+} channels. Blockade of these Ca^{2+} channels inhibits pain signal transmission by inhibiting the release of calcitonin gene-related peptide, glutamate, and substance P [39]. Ziconotide is one of the two medications approved by the FDA for the treatment of chronic pain in the IT space, and a number of clinical trials have shown that ziconotide is safe and efficacious in the treatment of intractable pain [40–43].

Significant adverse effects are associated with the administration of IT ziconotide at a sizable rate (11.6–30.6 % compared to a placebo rate of 2–10 %) and include psychiatric disturbances (depression, anxiety, hallucinations), pain, dizziness, diplopia, nystagmus, gait abnormalities, headache, cognitive (memory) impairment, speech disorder, urinary retention, nausea, somnolence, and nervousness [44–47].

The 2012 PACC considers ziconotide to be a treatment for patients with nociceptive and neuropathic pain. Ziconotide may be used alone as a first-line agent or in combination with an opioid as second-line treatment in the PACC algorithm. The use of ziconotide in combination with an opioid (hydromorphone or fentanyl), bupivacaine, or both opioid and bupivacaine was associated with delayed adverse effects leading to discontinuation of ziconotide in nearly two-thirds of the patients [48]. It should be noted that ziconotide has limited stability in combination with intrathecal morphine [49]. One must be cognizant that there is a higher prevalence of adverse effects associated with increased dosage, patient age, and titration rate [41]. Initial doses should not exceed 0.5–2.4 mcg/day and the maximum daily dose recommended is 19.2 mcg/day. Titration should be done carefully to limit the potential adverse effects.

Local Anesthetics (Bupivacaine)

Local anesthetics are commonly used in the treatment of both acute and chronic pain, and are utilized for both regional and neuraxial anesthesia. The mechanism of action for local anesthetics is to block the voltage-gated Na^+ channels in the neuronal cell membrane, thereby blocking action potential propagation [50]. Local anesthetics preferentially act on the fila radicularia given the large surface-to-volume ratio of the rootlets compared to the spinal cord [51].

Bupivacaine, an amide anesthetic with high lipid solubility, is the most commonly used local anesthetic utilized for continuous spinal infusion to relieve acute and chronic pain. Although many local anesthetics have been used for the treatment of pain in the IT space, bupivacaine is the only local anesthetic included in the PACC algorithms for IT therapies in neuropathic and nociceptive pain. According to the 2012 PACC algorithms, bupivacaine is considered to be first-line treatment in combination with morphine for neuropathic pain and second-line treatment for nociceptive pain in combination with opioids (fentanyl, hydromorphone, and morphine) [32]. Again, it should be noted that these recommendations are likely based on consensus rather than evidence, as local anesthetics block neuronal transmission of pain signals regardless of nociceptive or neuropathic nature. Combination therapy is often utilized because local anesthetics and opioids have been found to act synergistically when administered intrathecally for pain in acute pain (postoperative and labor) and animal models of chronic pain [52–58]. Combination therapy has the added benefit that it can also decrease the rate of dose escalation [37, 58]. Conversely, a double-blinded randomized control trial found that bupivacaine, up to 8 mg/day, did not offer better pain relief when added to opioids when compared to opioids alone [59]. However, other studies have shown a beneficial effect on pain with average bupivacaine daily doses around 10 mg [37, 60].

The long-term safety of bupivacaine infusion in the IT space has been shown in animal models [61, 62]. Although local anesthetics are considered to be safe, there is a potential for adverse effects such as neurotoxicity [63–65], weakness, numbness, urinary retention, and hypotension. The limiting factor is generally due to sensory and motor loss. Doses of IT bupivacaine as high as 125 mg/day have been reported [66]; however, guidelines recommend an initial dose of 1–4 mg/day and a maximum of 10 mg/day [32]. Nonetheless, many studies report average daily bupivacaine dosage around 10 mg [37, 60], suggesting that a substantial proportion of patients receive greater than 10 mg/day—especially if one factors in amounts received through patient-activated boluses.

Clonidine

Clonidine is a selective alpha-2 adrenergic agonist that is occasionally used in the spinal space for the treatment of pain. Clonidine acts by inhibiting nociceptive impulses at the dorsal horn of the spinal cord by activating pre- and post-junctional alpha-2 adrenoceptors. In addition to this mechanism, increasing evidence has shown that activated spinal cord glial cells contribute to enhanced pain states due to the release of proinflammatory cytokines. In the IT space, clonidine has been shown to markedly inhibit the neuroimmune activation associated with neuropathic pain states which is characterized by glial activation, production of cytokines, and activation of NF-κB and p38 [67].

The addition of clonidine may be considered for a patient who has neuropathic pain [32, 68–70] or to potentiate the effect of opioids, as alpha-2 agonists and opioids have a synergistic relationship [71–73]. According to the PACC 2012, clonidine may be used for neuropathic or nociceptive pain states. When treating neuropathic pain, it is a second-line agent when used with morphine or hydromorphone, a third-line agent as monotherapy or when used with fentanyl, and a fourth-line agent in combination with an opioid and/or bupivacaine. For nociceptive pain, it is a third-line agent when used in combination with an opioid and fourth line in combination with an opioid and bupivacaine. The starting dose recommended by the PACC is 40–100 mcg/day with a maximum recommended dose of 600 mcg/day [32]. It should be noted that clonidine has been shown to provide analgesia in a dose-dependent manner when used in the spinal space [67, 68, 74].

Adverse effects may include bradycardia, confusion, dizziness, dry mouth, hypotension, nausea, orthostasis, and sedation. Cardiovascular adverse effects paradoxically occur more frequently at lower doses. In addition, depression, insomnia, and night terrors have been reported with the use of intraspinal clonidine [75]. With abrupt discontinuation, rebound hypertension occurs [76], making titration down of clonidine, when used in combination with other drugs, a challenge.

Trialing

A trial is generally performed before a patient undergoes permanent implantation of an IDDS. The reasoning behind trialing is that it can provide clinical information on whether or not the therapy will prove to be efficacious for the patient. Although the trial only proves efficacy in the short term, the long-term efficacy can be inferred. There are many techniques that can be utilized when performing a trial. Trialing techniques include single shot or bolus dosing (epidural or IT), continuous infusions (epidural or IT), or using a combination of these methods. In addition, trialing can be performed on an inpatient or outpatient basis [77]. The most common technique utilized for trialing in the USA is the continuous IT catheter (45 %) [78]. The continuous IT catheter is considered to be the "gold standard" since it closely replicates the permanent IDDS. However, there is limited data to support that this technique is superior. One should also consider the potential disadvantages when placing a continuous catheter: risk of infection, increased cost, and the potential for spinal cord injury [79]. Additionally, most externalized pumps used in trialing deliver rates around 20 times the daily infusion rate used in IDDS; such high infusion rates result in wider and deeper spinal spread [24] and may explain occasional reports of significantly better analgesia during trial that are not replicated after implant. Each practitioner should adhere to a trialing protocol that is safe and appropriate to obtain the information needed to determine if a trial is successful or not. In general, a trial is considered successful if the patient has >50 % pain relief and at that point would undergo permanent implantation.

Clinical Application of an IDDS for Spine-Related Pain

FBSS and VCFs are the most common indications reported in the literature for IDDS use for spine-related pain [8, 11–13, 68, 80, 81]. FBSS refers to patients with persistent or new pain after spinal surgery for back or leg pain. In patients who have FBSS with a predominance of axial pain, an IDDS can be a good option if other more conservative measures fail or are not tolerated. Many studies have shown significant improvement in pain scores in FBSS patients following implant of an IDDS [8, 12–14]. VCFs can also cause a significant amount of axial pain amenable to treatment with an IDDS if refractory to conservative measures. In one study, 24 patients with severe osteoporosis and VCFs who were refractory to conservative measures underwent placement of an IDDS [9]. The results from this study by Shaladi et al. revealed significant improvement in VAS scores (8.7 pretrial to 1.9 at 12 months), improved quality of life/function, and eliminated use of oral opioids [9]. Although there is literature to support the use of IDDSs in patients with spine-related pain especially in patients with FBSS, there is a need for more supportive evidence with prospective randomized control trials.

Complications Associated with IDDS Implantation

The complications associated with IDDS implantation can be grouped into several categories which include drug, device, procedural, or programming related.

Drug complications are common and are most commonly associated with the use of IT opioids; these drug complications can include peripheral edema, hormonal changes, respiratory depression, and granuloma formation. IT ziconotide is associated with CNS side effects that may make the drug intolerable (see "Intrathecal Medications" for further discussion of drug complications). A retrospective review revealed that the most common cause of IDDS complication was secondary to IT medications, although the effects were transient (77 %) [82].

Complications due to the device can be attributed to the pump and/or the catheter. However, catheter-related complications do account for the majority of known device complications. Potential causes of device failure include changes in performance or failure of the catheter (micro-fracture, pinhole leak, kink, disconnection, breakage, shearing, migration, partial occlusion, tip fibrosis, inflammatory mass), unexpected battery depletion, component or motor failure (corrosion), and catheter access port failure [83]. One prospective study revealed that most catheter-related complications are determined by surgical technique [84]. The type of catheter used may also play a role in developing a potential complication [84]. Placement of the IT catheter in a paramedian approach can prevent shearing by spinous processes and decrease the likelihood of a catheter complication [82]. Device failure secondary to the pump is less common and has been reported to be between 1 and 12.5 % [82, 85]. Type of IT drug may play a role in device failure. Device failure has been reported to occur at a significantly higher rate when using non-approved IT drugs (7.0 %) versus approved IT drugs (2.4 %). Non-approved drugs can cause corrosion inside the pump due to corrosive agents (chloride ions, sulfate ions) in the drugs. Drug qualities such as hydrophobicity, degree of positive ionization, impurities, preservatives, pH adjustments, and concentration adjustments can increase the rate of corrosion. Catheter and device failure can result in abrupt cessation of IT medications and depending on the drug can be serious and potentially life threatening.

Procedural related complications include post-dural puncture headaches, CSF leak, pocket pain, spinal cord injury, hematomas (epidural or pocket), and wound dehiscence. Needle entry should be at or below the L2/3 interspace, if possible, to decrease the likelihood of spinal cord injury. Placement of a purse string suture around the catheter is recommended to reduce the chance of a CSF leak. Securing the reservoir to the fascia rather than the muscle will decrease the rate of persistent pocket pain. Adequate hemostasis and adherence to anticoagulation guidelines can help decrease the risk of hematoma. Should a patient develop a post-dural puncture headache, they can be managed conservatively with analgesics, hydration, caffeine, and laying in the supine position. If refractory, a post-dural puncture headache following IDDS placement may be treated with an epidural blood patch, and care must be taken to avoid damage to the IT catheter. Although there are many possible procedural complications, most can be avoided by utilizing proper surgical technique [34].

An IDDS-related infection is a potentially serious complication that may require discontinuation of therapy. The rate of infection reported in the literature is usually reported as less than 5 % [34]. A preoperative prevention technique for surgical site infection may include intranasal mupirocin in patients who are carriers of *Staphylococcus aureus* [86]. Some practitioners may have patients shower preoperatively with chlorhexidine gluconate which may reduce skin flora; however, it has not been found to reduce surgical site infections [87]. A superficial skin infection may be treated with close monitoring, consultation with an infectious disease specialist, and appropriate oral antibiotics. If a patient develops a deep infection the device should be removed, intraoperative cultures should be obtained, and appropriate antibiotics should be initiated. When an epidural or bony infection is suspected, advanced imaging with and without contrast should be ordered. There have been reports of successful device salvage, although this is not common practice and the risks and benefits must be weighed [88, 89].

Summary

IDDSs have proven to be beneficial in the treatment of chronic spine pain. When utilizing this treatment it is important to have in-depth knowledge of the neuraxial space, CSF flow dynamics, indications, IT medications, device matters, and potential complications. This advanced technology is not first-line therapy due to the fact it is invasive and costly, but when it is applied to a well-selected candidate it can be life changing. The current use of IDDSs focuses on chronic pain and spasticity although novel applications are being studied. Additionally, novel devices have entered the marked and some are in pre-market stages. The future of intrathecal drug delivery for pain will depend on successful delivery of positive outcomes with limited complications as well as on the performance of competing neurostimulation devices.

References

1. Brown J, et al. Disease-specific and generic health outcomes: a model for the evaluation of long-term intrathecal opioid therapy in noncancer low back pain patients. Clin J Pain. 1999;15(2):122–31.
2. Deer TR, et al. Polyanalgesic Consensus Conference 2012: recommendations for the management of pain by intrathecal (intraspinal) drug delivery: report of an interdisciplinary expert panel. Neuromodulation. 2012;15(5):436–64. discussion 464–6.
3. Hayek SM, et al. Age-dependent intrathecal opioid escalation in chronic noncancer pain patients. Pain Med. 2011;12(8):1179–89.

4. Rauck RL, et al. Long-term intrathecal opioid therapy with a patient-activated, implanted delivery system for the treatment of refractory cancer pain. J Pain. 2003;4(8):441–7.
5. Smith TJ, et al. Randomized clinical trial of an implantable drug delivery system compared with comprehensive medical management for refractory cancer pain: impact on pain, drug-related toxicity, and survival. J Clin Oncol. 2002;20(19):4040–9.
6. Onofrio BM, Yaksh TL. Long-term pain relief produced by intrathecal morphine infusion in 53 patients. J Neurosurg. 1990;72(2):200–9.
7. Penn RD, Paice JA. Chronic intrathecal morphine for intractable pain. J Neurosurg. 1987;67(2):182–6.
8. Atli A, et al. Intrathecal opioid therapy for chronic nonmalignant pain: a retrospective cohort study with 3-year follow-up. Pain Med. 2010;11(7):1010–6.
9. Shaladi A, et al. Continuous intrathecal morphine infusion in patients with vertebral fractures due to osteoporosis. Clin J Pain. 2007;23(6):511–7.
10. Deer T, et al. Intrathecal drug delivery for treatment of chronic low back pain: report from the National Outcomes Registry for Low Back Pain. Pain Med. 2004;5(1):6–13.
11. Rainov NG, Heidecke V, Burkert W. Long-term intrathecal infusion of drug combinations for chronic back and leg pain. J Pain Symptom Manage. 2001;22(4):862–71.
12. Anderson VC, Burchiel KJ. A prospective study of long-term intrathecal morphine in the management of chronic nonmalignant pain. Neurosurgery. 1999;44(2):289–300. discussion 300–1.
13. Roberts LJ, et al. Outcome of intrathecal opioids in chronic non-cancer pain. Eur J Pain. 2001;5(4):353–61.
14. Winkelmuller M, Winkelmuller W. Long-term effects of continuous intrathecal opioid treatment in chronic pain of nonmalignant etiology. J Neurosurg. 1996;85(3):458–67.
15. Battal B, et al. Cerebrospinal fluid flow imaging by using phase-contrast MR technique. Br J Radiol. 2011;84(1004):758–65.
16. Greitz D, Franck A, Nordell B. On the pulsatile nature of intracranial and spinal CSF-circulation demonstrated by MR imaging. Acta Radiol. 1993;34(4):321–8.
17. Enzmann DR, Pelc NJ. Normal flow patterns of intracranial and spinal cerebrospinal fluid defined with phase-contrast cine MR imaging. Radiology. 1991;178(2):467–74.
18. Greitz D. Cerebrospinal fluid circulation and associated intracranial dynamics. A radiologic investigation using MR imaging and radionuclide cisternography. Acta Radiol Suppl. 1993;386:1–23.
19. Henry-Feugeas MC, et al. Origin of subarachnoid cerebrospinal fluid pulsations: a phase-contrast MR analysis. Magn Reson Imaging. 2000;18(4):387–95.
20. Friese S, et al. The influence of pulse and respiration on spinal cerebrospinal fluid pulsation. Invest Radiol. 2004;39(2):120–30.
21. Alperin N, et al. Hemodynamically independent analysis of cerebrospinal fluid and brain motion observed with dynamic phase contrast MRI. Magn Reson Med. 1996;35(5):741–54.
22. Grider JS, Harned ME, Etscheidt MA. Patient selection and outcomes using a low-dose intrathecal opioid trialing method for chronic nonmalignant pain. Pain Physician. 2011;14(4):343–51.
23. Yamada S, et al. Influence of respiration on cerebrospinal fluid movement using magnetic resonance spin labeling. Fluids Barriers CNS. 2013;10(1):36.
24. Bernards CM. Cerebrospinal fluid and spinal cord distribution of baclofen and bupivacaine during slow intrathecal infusion in pigs. Anesthesiology. 2006;105(1):169–78.
25. Flack SH, Anderson CM, Bernards C. Morphine distribution in the spinal cord after chronic infusion in pigs. Anesth Analg. 2011;112(2):460–4.
26. Alperin N, et al. MRI study of cerebral blood flow and CSF flow dynamics in an upright posture: the effect of posture on the intracranial compliance and pressure. Acta Neurochir Suppl. 2005;95:177–81.
27. Hocking G, Wildsmith JA. Intrathecal drug spread. Br J Anaesth. 2004;93(4):568–78.

28. Yaksh TL, et al. Analgesia produced by a spinal action of morphine and effects upon parturition in the rat. Anesthesiology. 1979;51(5):386–92.
29. Krames ES. Intraspinal opioid therapy for chronic nonmalignant pain: current practice and clinical guidelines. J Pain Symptom Manage. 1996;11(6):333–52.
30. Sylvester RK, Lindsay SM, Schauer C. The conversion challenge: from intrathecal to oral morphine. Am J Hosp Palliat Care. 2004;21(2):143–7.
31. Kroin JS. Intrathecal drug administration. Present use and future trends. Clin Pharmacokinet. 1992;22(5):319–26.
32. Deer TR. Polyanalgesic Consensus Conference 2012. Neuromodulation. 2012;15(5):418–9.
33. Hamza M, et al. Prospective study of 3-year follow-up of low-dose intrathecal opioids in the management of chronic nonmalignant pain. Pain Med. 2012;13(10):1304–13.
34. Deer TR, et al. Polyanalgesic Consensus Conference–2012: recommendations to reduce morbidity and mortality in intrathecal drug delivery in the treatment of chronic pain. Neuromodulation. 2012;15(5):467–82. discussion 482.
35. Deer TR, et al. Polyanalgesic Consensus Conference–2012: consensus on diagnosis, detection, and treatment of catheter-tip granulomas (inflammatory masses). Neuromodulation. 2012;15(5):483–95. discussion 496.
36. Allen JW, et al. Opiate pharmacology of intrathecal granulomas. Anesthesiology. 2006;105(3):590–8.
37. Veizi IE, et al. Combination of intrathecal opioids with bupivacaine attenuates opioid dose escalation in chronic noncancer pain patients. Pain Med. 2011;12(10):1481–9.
38. De Andres J, et al. Can an intrathecal, catheter-tip-associated inflammatory mass reoccur? Clin J Pain. 2010;26(7):631–4.
39. McGivern JG. Ziconotide: a review of its pharmacology and use in the treatment of pain. Neuropsychiatr Dis Treat. 2007;3(1):69–85.
40. Jain KK. An evaluation of intrathecal ziconotide for the treatment of chronic pain. Expert Opin Investig Drugs. 2000;9(10):2403–10.
41. Rauck RL, et al. A randomized, double-blind, placebo-controlled study of intrathecal ziconotide in adults with severe chronic pain. J Pain Symptom Manage. 2006;31(5):393–406.
42. Wallace MS, et al. Intrathecal ziconotide in the treatment of chronic nonmalignant pain: a randomized, double-blind, placebo-controlled clinical trial. Neuromodulation. 2006;9(2):75–86.
43. Staats PS, et al. Intrathecal ziconotide in the treatment of refractory pain in patients with cancer or AIDS: a randomized controlled trial. JAMA. 2004;291(1):63–70.
44. Wallace MS, et al. Intrathecal ziconotide for severe chronic pain: safety and tolerability results of an open-label, long-term trial. Anesth Analg. 2008;106(2):628–37, table of contents.
45. Webster LR, et al. Long-term intrathecal ziconotide for chronic pain: an open-label study. J Pain Symptom Manage. 2009;37(3):363–72.
46. Kapural L, et al. Intrathecal ziconotide for complex regional pain syndrome: seven case reports. Pain Pract. 2009;9(4):296–303.
47. Rauck RL, et al. Intrathecal ziconotide for neuropathic pain: a review. Pain Pract. 2009;9(5):327–37.
48. Hayek SM, et al. Ziconotide combination intrathecal therapy for noncancer pain is limited secondary to delayed adverse effects: a case series with a 24-month follow-up. Neuromodulation. 2015;18(5):397–403.
49. Shields DEP, Aclan JB, Szatkowski AB. Chemical stability of admixtures containing ziconotide 25 mcg/mL and morphine sulfate 10 mg/mL or 20 mg/mL during simulated intrathecal administration. Int J Pharm Compd. 2008;12(6):553–7.
50. Butterworth 4th JF, Strichartz GR. Molecular mechanisms of local anesthesia: a review. Anesthesiology. 1990;72(4):711–34.
51. Boswell MV, Iacono RP, Guthkelch AN. Sites of action of subarachnoid lidocaine and tetracaine: observations with evoked potential monitoring during spinal cord stimulator implantation. Reg Anesth. 1992;17(1):37–42.

52. Tejwani GA, Rattan AK, McDonald JS. Role of spinal opioid receptors in the antinociceptive interactions between intrathecal morphine and bupivacaine. Anesth Analg. 1992;74(5):726–34.
53. Penning JP, Yaksh TL. Interaction of intrathecal morphine with bupivacaine and lidocaine in the rat. Anesthesiology. 1992;77(6):1186–2000.
54. Ortner CM, et al. On the ropivacaine-reducing effect of low-dose sufentanil in intrathecal labor analgesia. Acta Anaesthesiol Scand. 2010;54(8):1000–6.
55. Parpaglioni R, et al. Adding sufentanil to levobupivacaine or ropivacaine intrathecal anaesthesia affects the minimum local anaesthetic dose required. Acta Anaesthesiol Scand. 2009;53(9):1214–20.
56. Nitescu P, et al. Continuous infusion of opioid and bupivacaine by externalized intrathecal catheters in long-term treatment of "refractory" nonmalignant pain. Clin J Pain. 1998;14(1):17–28.
57. Chestnut DH, et al. Continuous infusion epidural analgesia during labor: a randomized, double-blind comparison of 0.0625 % bupivacaine/0.0002 % fentanyl versus 0.125 % bupivacaine. Anesthesiology. 1988;68(5):754–9.
58. van Dongen RT, Crul BJ, van Egmond J. Intrathecal coadministration of bupivacaine diminishes morphine dose progression during long-term intrathecal infusion in cancer patients. Clin J Pain. 1999;15(3):166–72.
59. Mironer YE, et al. Efficacy and safety of intrathecal opioid/bupivacaine mixture in chronic nonmalignant pain: a double blind, randomized, crossover, multicenter study by the National Forum of Independent Pain Clinicians (NFIPC). Neuromodulation. 2002;5(4):208–13.
60. Deer TR, et al. Clinical experience with intrathecal bupivacaine in combination with opioid for the treatment of chronic pain related to failed back surgery syndrome and metastatic cancer pain of the spine. Spine J. 2002;2(4):274–8.
61. Kroin JS, et al. The effect of chronic subarachnoid bupivacaine infusion in dogs. Anesthesiology. 1987;66(6):737–42.
62. Li DF, et al. Neurological toxicity of the subarachnoid infusion of bupivacaine, lignocaine or 2-chloroprocaine in the rat. Br J Anaesth. 1985;57(4):424–9.
63. Zhong Z, et al. Repeated intrathecal administration of ropivacaine causes neurotoxicity in rats. Anaesth Intensive Care. 2009;37(6):929–36.
64. Yang SH, Guo QL, Wang YC. Alterations of myelin basic protein concentration in the plasma and ultrastructure in the spinal cord after continuous intrathecal ropivacaine injection in rats. Zhong Nan Da Xue Xue Bao Yi Xue Ban. 2008;33(6):527–32.
65. Yamashita A, et al. A comparison of the neurotoxic effects on the spinal cord of tetracaine, lidocaine, bupivacaine, and ropivacaine administered intrathecally in rabbits. Anesth Analg. 2003;97(2):512–9, table of contents.
66. Lundborg C, et al. Clinical experience using intrathecal (IT) bupivacaine infusion in three patients with complex regional pain syndrome type I (CRPS-I). Acta Anaesthesiol Scand. 1999;43(6):667–78.
67. Feng X, et al. Intrathecal administration of clonidine attenuates spinal neuroimmune activation in a rat model of neuropathic pain with existing hyperalgesia. Eur J Pharmacol. 2009;614(1–3):38–43.
68. Eisenach JC, Hood DD, Curry R. Intrathecal, but not intravenous, clonidine reduces experimental thermal or capsaicin-induced pain and hyperalgesia in normal volunteers. Anesth Analg. 1998;87(3):591–6.
69. Uhle EI, et al. Continuous intrathecal clonidine administration for the treatment of neuropathic pain. Stereotact Funct Neurosurg. 2000;75(4):167–75.
70. Siddall PJ, et al. Intrathecal morphine and clonidine in the management of spinal cord injury pain: a case report. Pain. 1994;59(1):147–8.
71. Sites BD, et al. Intrathecal clonidine added to a bupivacaine-morphine spinal anesthetic improves postoperative analgesia for total knee arthroplasty. Anesth Analg. 2003;96(4):1083–8, table of contents.

72. Mogensen T, et al. Epidural clonidine enhances postoperative analgesia from a combined low-dose epidural bupivacaine and morphine regimen. Anesth Analg. 1992;75(4):607–10.
73. Capogna G, et al. Addition of clonidine to epidural morphine enhances postoperative analgesia after cesarean delivery. Reg Anesth. 1995;20(1):57–61.
74. Hao JX, et al. Effects of intrathecal vs. systemic clonidine in treating chronic allodynia-like response in spinally injured rats. Brain Res. 1996;736(1–2):28–34.
75. Bevacqua BK, Fattouh M, Backonja M. Depression, night terrors, and insomnia associated with long-term intrathecal clonidine therapy. Pain Pract. 2007;7(1):36–8.
76. Fitzgibbon D, et al. Rebound hypertension and withdrawal associated with discontinuation of an infusion of epidural clonidine. Anesthesiology. 1996;84(3):729–31.
77. Deer TR, et al. Polyanalgesic Consensus Conference–2012: recommendations on trialing for intrathecal (intraspinal) drug delivery: report of an interdisciplinary expert panel. Neuromodulation. 2012;15(5):420–35. discussion 435.
78. Ahmed SU, Martin NM, Chang Y. Patient selection and trial methods for intraspinal drug delivery for chronic pain: a national survey. Neuromodulation. 2005;8(2):112–20.
79. Anderson VC, Burchiel KJ, Cooke B. A prospective, randomized trial of intrathecal injection vs. epidural infusion in the selection of patients for continuous intrathecal opioid therapy. Neuromodulation. 2003;6(3):142–52.
80. Doleys DM, Brown JL, Ness T. Multidimensional outcomes analysis of intrathecal, oral opioid, and behavioral-functional restoration therapy for failed back surgery syndrome: a retrospective study with 4 years' follow-up. Neuromodulation. 2006;9(4):270–83.
81. Ilias W, et al. Patient-controlled analgesia in chronic pain patients: experience with a new device designed to be used with implanted programmable pumps. Pain Pract. 2008;8(3):164–70.
82. Kamran S, Wright BD. Complications of intrathecal drug delivery systems. Neuromodulation. 2001;4(3):111–5.
83. Jones RL, Rawlins PK. The diagnosis of intrathecal infusion pump system failure. Pain Physician. 2005;8(3):291–6.
84. Follett KA, Naumann CP. A prospective study of catheter-related complications of intrathecal drug delivery systems. J Pain Symptom Manage. 2000;19(3):209–15.
85. Fluckiger B, et al. Device-related complications of long-term intrathecal drug therapy via implanted pumps. Spinal Cord. 2008;46(9):639–43.
86. Kallen AJ, Wilson CT, Larson RJ. Perioperative intranasal mupirocin for the prevention of surgical-site infections: systematic review of the literature and meta-analysis. Infect Control Hosp Epidemiol. 2005;26(12):916–22.
87. Webster J, Osborne S. Preoperative bathing or showering with skin antiseptics to prevent surgical site infection. Cochrane Database Syst Rev. 2015;2, CD004985.
88. Peerdeman SM, de Groot V, Feller RE. In situ treatment of an infected intrathecal baclofen pump implant with gentamicin-impregnated collagen fleece. J Neurosurg. 2010;112(6):1308–10.
89. Diefenbeck M, Muckley T, Hofmann GO. Prophylaxis and treatment of implant-related infections by local application of antibiotics. Injury. 2006;37 Suppl 2:S95–104.

Part IV
Surgical Pain Therapies

Chapter 15
Epidural Paddle Placement for Spinal Cord Stimulation

Peter G. Campbell and Steven M. Falowski

Key Points

- Spine surgeons are required to place a paddle electrode array via laminectomy or laminotomy.
- Implantation of a permanent system involving paddle electrode is typically considered after the completion of a successful external trial with a percutaneously placed lead.
- Paddle electrode implantation may be performed either under monitored anesthesia care or under general anesthesia.
- Multiple arrays or different electrode configurations can be constructed with paddle electrodes. They are more energy efficient and have the advantage of current steering, as well as current shielding.
- An advantage of paddle electrodes resides in their more inherent stability in the dorsal epidural space and lesser propensity to migrate.
- Preoperative MRI imaging of the area of electrode insertion is recommended.

P.G. Campbell, M.D. (✉)
Division of Neurosurgery, Parkway Neuroscience and Spine Institute,
17 Western Maryland Parkway, Hagerstown, MD 21795, USA
e-mail: pcampbell@pnsi.org

S.M. Falowski, M.D.
Neurosurgery, St. Luke's University Health Network,
701 Ostrum St, Suite 302, Bethlehem, PA 18017, USA
e-mail: sfalowski@gmail.com

© Springer International Publishing Switzerland 2016
S.M. Falowski, J.E. Pope (eds.), *Integrating Pain Treatment into Your Spine Practice*, DOI 10.1007/978-3-319-27796-7_15

Introduction

Spinal cord stimulation (SCS) is a widely used, effective modality for treating chronic pain. In the USA, the most common indication for SCS is failed back surgery [1, 2]. Other indications include lumbosacral radiculopathy and complex regional pain syndromes [3]. The efficacy of this technique has been demonstrated in several sizeable studies when offered as a comparison with best medical management, as well as a revision surgical procedure [2, 4, 5].

Proceeding with the implantation of a permanent system involving an epidural paddle electrode array and a subcutaneous pulse generator typically is only considered after the completion of a successful external trial with a percutaneously placed lead. However, there are situations in which an open paddle electrode trial is performed such as with previous thoracic spinal surgery or when a percutaneous lead cannot be placed whether secondary to scar tissue in the epidural space or inability to enter the epidural space secondary to bony fusion. While placement of permanent percutaneous system is an option, many authors report the longevity of the pain relief is inferior to a paddle based system owing to the increased incidence of postoperative lead migration [2, 6–8]. In either condition, the anatomic location chosen for conclusive lead placement is based on the information accumulated from the trial. The permanent lead is secured in a position so that the contacts of the permanent electrode cover all the areas of the active and beneficial electrode contacts during the trial and thus result in coverage in the identical somatic locations as the trial electrode [9].

Spinal cord stimulation has been used to treat patients with a wide range of pain syndromes including failed back syndrome, peripheral artery disease, refractory angina, diabetic neuropathy, post-herpetic neuralgia, post-amputation pain, and complex regional pain syndrome [10]. Accordingly, the use in multidisciplinary spine and pain clinics continues to expand. Oftentimes, spine surgeons are asked to place a paddle electrode array via laminectomy for treatment of one of these maladies. This chapter attempts to discuss the procedural planning and operative technique associated with such implants.

Paddle Electrodes

Multiple arrays or different electrode configurations can be constructed with paddle electrodes. The main advantage of paddle electrodes resides in their stability in the dorsal epidural space and lesser propensity to migrate. Some data by North also suggest a broader stimulation pattern and lower stimulation requirements with paddle electrodes which leads to more energy efficiency in delivering electrical stimulation [7]. Another advantage is the ease in current steering, as well as current shielding.

Paddle electrodes come in many configurations and sizes. There are single and dual column electrodes available from all manufacturers, as well as Tripole configurations available from Medtronic Inc and St. Jude Medical Inc. There are four column paddle electrodes from Boston Scientific Inc, as well as the Pentad electrode available from St. Jude Medical Inc.

There are inherent benefits in paddle electrode placement. North et al. have published on comparison between plate and percutaneous electrode placement. Although more invasive than percutaneous placement, paddle placement yielded significantly better clinical results in patients with failed back surgery syndrome at up to 3 year follow-up [6, 7]. The evidence also demonstrated that shaping of the electrical field is possible with paddle electrodes leading to more complex electrode arrays and stimulation configurations [6]. Holsheimer et al. examined tripole configurations demonstrating the ability to have finer control of paresthesia [11]. Electrical field steering could change the paresthesia area completely. When the transverse tripolar configurations are used the threshold for stimulation of dorsal roots is higher, compared with the dorsal column threshold. This results in a wider therapeutic range, wider paresthesia coverage, and a greater probability to fully cover the painful area with paresthesia. This leads to the concepts of enhanced current steering and current shielding yielding to innumerable available programming configurations [12, 13].

Preoperative Planning

Evaluating any patient's surgical candidacy must involve deliberation into the condition, patient-specific risk analysis, and a benefit advantage of the procedure. Consideration of underlying medical comorbidities and anticoagulant use may require the input of other specialists including primary care, cardiology, or pulmonology prior to proceeding with a prone surgical procedure that will require abstention from anticoagulants and antiplatelet agents. Exclusion criteria for SCS implantation include an uncontrolled psychiatric disorder, persistent local or systemic infection, immunosuppression, and anticoagulant or antiplatelet therapy that cannot be suspended [14]. Only once these preoperative conditions have been satisfied can surgical planning commence.

An open paddle electrode implant may be performed either under monitored anesthesia care which allows for intraoperative real time trial stimulation or under general anesthesia which precludes patient interaction during surgery [15]. Some authors have advocated some novel minimal access approaches to paddle placement to allow the procedure to be performed under monitored anesthesia care or even spinal anesthesia [16, 17]. Oftentimes, in the setting of morbid obesity, obstructive sleep apnea, or chronic obstructive pulmonary disease many anesthesiologists prefer a general anesthetic secondary to the risks of hypoxia while prone [18]. Also, many patients cannot participate with an awake procedure secondary to various concerns such as language barriers, cognitive issues, and occasionally revision procedures requiring operative times of longer duration. Furthermore, in cases of cervical paddle placement, general anesthesia is typically desired for patient safety and the ability to temporarily fixate the craniocervical junction in a point of maximum flexion that would not be otherwise possible [19]. In a previous report, asleep stimulator placement was associated with an improved outcome over the awake cohort [15]. At present, the authors routinely perform implantation of paddle electrodes under general anesthesia. Electrophysiological monitoring relating to the spinal segment of interest with SSEP and EMG recording is utilized. To compensate for variability of physiologic midline, multi-column paddle electrodes are employed. The correct cephalocaudal placement is determined from the stimulation during the percutaneous trial.

For paddle electrode placement there is some debate as to the value of obtaining a preoperative MRI of the area of interest prior to implant. While the authors are not aware of any published retrospective evaluation regarding the necessity of this imaging preoperatively, many spine surgeons do advocate preoperative MRI, especially when implanting in the cervical spine given the smaller diameter of the canal at that location. There is a case series in the literature whereby large disc herniations at T6/7, T7/8, and T8/9 were the likely causative factor of an irreversible lower extremity paralysis after SCS implant [20]. A commenter to this report suggested preoperative imaging would have avoided this complication [21]. It is the authors' practice to perform an MRI of the desired region, whether cervical or thoracic in every case.

Open Thoracic Epidural Electrode Array Placement

After preoperative planning and determination of the anesthetic regimen the first step in the surgical procedure is proper positioning of the patient. The prone position is typically utilized unless the there is a plan to place the generator in the anterior abdominal region. In that case the lateral position may be utilized. Bed selection is institution dependent. For thoracic epidural paddle placement many implanters may use the Jackson spinal table as these cases are often integrated into the operative caseload of degenerative spinal conditions that also are treated on this table. Other authors describe the use of either bolsters or a radiolucent Wilson frame [22]. The C-Arm should be positioned to provide a true anterior-posterior view. It is imperative that the spinous process be aligned in the middle of the field with the endplates aligned at the region of interest to ensure accuracy. The level of ideal stimulation and target coverage in the spine should be determined from the trial and can be anatomically confirmed by rib counting on the AP view. The author will typically place a radiopaque marker on what is thought to be the pedicle of the 11th vertebrae during the trial electrode placement in order to provide a frame of reference for the paddle implant.

After positioning, draping and level confirmation, exposure to the segment of interest is performed via incision and subperiosteal dissection down to the lamina. The thoracic incision is typically made a spinal level below the location at which the paddle lead is to be placed. The author utilizes a low profile, frame-based retractor system with transverse ratcheting retractor bodies for exposure similar to that used for anterior cervical exposure. Other retractors utilized may include a cerebellar retractor or Williams retractor. Once exposure has been achieved, a laminotomy or laminectomy should be performed to provide access to the level of interest. Some authors advocate electrode placement through a tubular retraction system to reduce length of stay [23]. There are also reports of placement via unilateral laminotomy [17]. Nevertheless, sufficient bone should be removed so as not to limit the angle of introduction of the electrode [22]. After bone removal with a high speed drill, 2 mm Kerrison rongeurs are used to expose the spinal canal and remove the ligamentum flavum.

After exposure and laminotomy has been performed, care must be taken when placing instruments in the dorsal epidural space of the unprotected spinal cord as any ventrally directed force may result in neurologic injury. There are limited options to free the epidural space along the entire course of the electrode. The tool most commonly utilized is a Woodson dural separator for this purpose. Subsequent to preparing the epidural space, the electrode template is then passed cranially in the epidural space while maintaining attention to any ventral force vectors so as to avoid compressing the spinal cord. It is the authors' recommendation to place the template and/or electrode with a force parallel to the spinal cord to limit the risk of spinal cord compression and subsequent injury. It is therefore imperative to employ methods to decrease the angle of incidence with the spinal cord. If the paddle will not advance after this exposure there are several options. There have been reports of the use of a malleable wire snare suture retriever to assist with electrode steerage [24]. Another technique that the authors find consistently helpful is the creation of a 1.5–2 mm trough, spanning the entire length of the lamina to provide access for a blunt nerve hook in an effort to break up dural adhesions that are not allowing midline paddle electrode placement [25]. The last resort in the setting of an electrode not passing to the desired location is performing another laminotomy or laminectomy at a higher level to create more space and access for safe electrode introduction [22]. In the thoracic spine the leads are often tethered with stress relaxation loops or via anchors sutured to the paraspinal musculature with the leads passed percutaneously to the battery site (Fig. 15.1). The author finds it useful to leave a portion of ligamentum flavum attached to the subjacent lamina for the purpose of lead stabilization with either a butterfly anchor or suture.

Lead migration and infection are common forms of spinal cord stimulator failure [26]. Rates of paddle migration vary between series from 3 to 32 % [27]. However, as hardware technology has improved over the years, current reports show rates approaching zero for the indication of spontaneous fracture, migration, or infection after thoracic epidural paddle electrode array implant [28]. Even with the successes gained by implant improvements, most studies continue to report about one-third of implanted patients become non-responders to long-term SCS therapy [28]. In the authors' experience this typically occurs within the first 2 years after implant. Accordingly, some of these patients will occasionally request hardware removal secondary to lack of efficacy. Thus, revision and removal of the epidural electrode array can be performed safely if adherence to the dorsal plane of scar tissue surrounding the lead is incised and removed [29].

Fig. 15.1 Intraoperative
fluoroscopic image
showing a thoracic multi
column paddle electrode
covering the entire
vertebral body of T9 with
some coverage over the
T8/T9 disc space

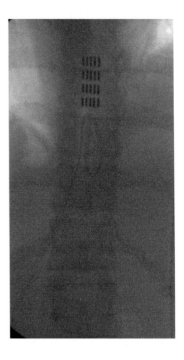

Open Cervical Epidural Electrode Array Placement

Neuromodulation via cervical stimulation is often utilized to control neck and upper
extremity pain. In order to obtain coverage in the neck and upper extremity, an
upper cervical vertebral body is typically targeted. However, some authors' enthu-
siasm for cervical spinal cord stimulation is tempered by the challenge of securing
an electrode in this inherently more flexible region [30]. Unsurprisingly, there is
reportedly a higher rate of lead migration in the cervical spine than the thoracic
spine [31]. Additionally, preoperative imaging with cervical MRI is more critical in
this region leading some authors to uniformly recommend it preoperatively [32].
The authors always obtain an MRI prior to paddle implant in order to assess canal
diameter so an appropriately sized paddle may be selected. The authors perform the
procedure under general anesthesia with the head stabilized in a Mayfield head
frame so as to obtain maximum flexion and temporary reversal of the cervical lor-
dosis. However, there are reports in the literature of this procedure being done under
conscious sedation with good results [33].

Two options exist for the passage of a paddle electrode in this spinal segment.
Anterograde cervical epidural paddle electrode placement is possible only after
laminotomy or laminectomy. Placing a high cervical epidural paddle in the cephalad
direction certainly offers benefits in terms of operative ease [29]. Fluoroscopy is
used to plan the skin incision which is generally about 5 cm in length. Typically, the
laminotomy is performed at the C4/5 or C5/6 interspace depending on paddle length.
The electrode is then advanced under fluoroscopic guidance to the planned level.

If any epidural resistance hinders electrode placement, additional laminotomies are performed and a more extensive epidural dissection is carried out so adhesions can be separated under direct visualization [33].

If a retrograde paddle placement is desired, the patient is positioned prone in pins with capital flexion. Two techniques have been described for retrograde paddle placement. The most frequently reported technique involves placement at C1/C2, while newer reports demonstrate feasibility of placement at C0/C1 [32–34]. Incision is made from the occiput down to C2 or C3. At that point either a laminotomy at C1 to expose the epidural plane for C1/2 retrograde passage or blunt dissection of the posterior occipito-atlantic membrane to find the dural plane superior to the level of C1 is performed. Subsequently, the spinal cord electrode is then advanced in a retrograde fashion under fluoroscopy to its ideal position.

Given the flexion in the region special attention is typically paid to securing the electrode in place. Most authors strongly suggest a sizeable stress relaxation loop in the cervical region [27, 32–34]. Some recommend anchor placement with suture to the paraspinal musculature [32]. Papahill reports a 0 % lead migration rate with "several" strain relief loops of electrode placed deep to the subfascial with no additional anchoring [33]. The authors tend to place sizeable stress relaxation loops in both the cervical region and at the battery insertion site as to alleviate any points of increased strain along the system. Care is taken to ensure the leads are tunneled out of the cervical spine in a submuscular and subfascial manner. Given the higher rates of migration in the cervical spine, utilizing good surgical technique at implant date almost certainly decreases the rate of postoperative lead migration.

Summary

Both the hardware and software utilized in the treatment of chronic pain by spinal cord stimulation continue to improve. Manufacturers have improved paddle electrodes and leads, thereby markedly decreasing the rate of spontaneous lead fracture and migration [28]. New paradigms of stimulation such as burst and high-frequency tonic programing are being applied at the software level in order to provide paresthesia free coverage with many patients finding better pain relief and improved pain quality through these modalities [35]. Given the current array of implant choices and the emerging technologies that are certain to be released in the near future, the options available for neuromodulation will continue to offer providers even more flexibility with an ever expanding set of indications for treatment of chronic pain.

References

1. North RB, Kidd D, Shipley J, Taylor RS. Spinal cord stimulation versus reoperation for failed back surgery syndrome: a cost effectiveness and cost utility analysis based on a randomized, controlled trial. Neurosurgery. 2007;61(2):361–8. discussion 68–9.

2. North RB, Kidd DH, Farrokhi F, Piantadosi SA. Spinal cord stimulation versus repeated lumbosacral spine surgery for chronic pain: a randomized, controlled trial. Neurosurgery. 2005;56(1):98–106. discussion 06–7.

3. Lee AW, Pilitsis JG. Spinal cord stimulation: indications and outcomes. Neurosurg Focus. 2006;21(6), E3.

4. Kumar K, Taylor RS, Jacques L, Eldabe S, Meglio M, Molet J, et al. Spinal cord stimulation versus conventional medical management for neuropathic pain: a multicentre randomised controlled trial in patients with failed back surgery syndrome. Pain. 2007;132(1–2):179–88.

5. Kumar K, Taylor RS, Jacques L, Eldabe S, Meglio M, Molet J, et al. The effects of spinal cord stimulation in neuropathic pain are sustained: a 24-month follow-up of the prospective randomized controlled multicenter trial of the effectiveness of spinal cord stimulation. Neurosurgery. 2008;63(4):762–70. discussion 70.

6. North RB, Kidd DH, Petrucci L, Dorsi MJ. Spinal cord stimulation electrode design: a prospective, randomized, controlled trial comparing percutaneous with laminectomy electrodes: part II-clinical outcomes. Neurosurgery. 2005;57(5):990–6. discussion 90–6.

7. North RB, Kidd DH, Olin JC, Sieracki JM. Spinal cord stimulation electrode design: prospective, randomized, controlled trial comparing percutaneous and laminectomy electrodes-part I: technical outcomes. Neurosurgery. 2002;51(2):381–9. discussion 89–90.

8. North RB, Kidd D, Davis C, Olin J, Sieracki JM. Spinal cord stimulation electrode design: a prospective randomized, controlled trial comparing percutaneous and laminectomy electrodes. Stereotact Funct Neurosurg. 1999;73(1–4):134.

9. Mammis A, Mogilner AY. The use of intraoperative electrophysiology for the placement of spinal cord stimulator paddle leads under general anesthesia. Neurosurgery. 2012;70(2 Suppl Operative):230–6.

10. Deer TR, Thomson S, Pope JE, Russo M, Luscombe F, Levy R. International neuromodulation society critical assessment: guideline review of implantable neurostimulation devices. Neuromodulation. 2014;17(7):678–85. discussion 85.

11. Holsheimer J, Nuttin B, King GW, Wesselink WA, Gybels JM, de Sutter P. Clinical evaluation of paresthesia steering with a new system for spinal cord stimulation. Neurosurgery. 1998;42(3):541–7. discussion 47–9.

12. Falowski S, Celii A, Sharan A. Spinal cord stimulation: an update. Neurotherapeutics. 2008;5(1):86–99.

13. Falowski S, Sharan A. A review on spinal cord stimulation. J Neurosurg Sci. 2012;56(4):287–98.

14. North RB, Kidd DH, Olin J, Sieracki JM, Boulay M. Spinal cord stimulation with interleaved pulses: a randomized, controlled trial. Neuromodulation. 2007;10(4):349–57.

15. Falowski SM, Celii A, Sestokas AK, Schwartz DM, Matsumoto C, Sharan A. Awake vs. asleep placement of spinal cord stimulators: a cohort analysis of complications associated with placement. Neuromodulation. 2011;14(2):130–4. discussion 34–5.

16. Sarubbo S, Latini F, Tugnoli V, Quatrale R, Granieri E, Cavallo MA. Spinal anesthesia and minimal invasive laminotomy for paddle electrode placement in spinal cord stimulation: technical report and clinical results at long-term followup. ScientificWorldJournal. 2012;2012:201053.

17. Vangeneugden J. Implantation of surgical electrodes for spinal cord stimulation: classical midline laminotomy technique versus minimal invasive unilateral technique combined with spinal anaesthesia. Acta Neurochir Suppl. 2007;97(Pt 1):111–4.

18. Air EL, Toczyl GR, Mandybur GT. Electrophysiologic monitoring for placement of laminectomy leads for spinal cord stimulation under general anesthesia. Neuromodulation. 2012;15(6):573–9. discussion 79–80.

19. Balzer JR, Tomycz ND, Crammond DJ, Habeych M, Thirumala PD, Urgo L, et al. Localization of cervical and cervicomedullary stimulation leads for pain treatment using median nerve somatosensory evoked potential collision testing. J Neurosurg. 2011;114(1):200–5.

20. Smith CC, Lin JL, Shokat M, Dosanjh SS, Casthely D. A report of paraparesis following spinal cord stimulator trial, implantation and revision. Pain Physician. 2010;13(4):357–63.

21. Gilbert JW, Wheeler GR, Mick GE, Herder SL, Richardson GB. Paraparesis following spinal cord stimulator trial, implantation and revision. Pain Physician. 2010;13(6), E377.
22. Levy R, Henderson J, Slavin K, Simpson BA, Barolat G, Shipley J, et al. Incidence and avoidance of neurologic complications with paddle type spinal cord stimulation leads. Neuromodulation. 2011;14(5):412–22. discussion 22.
23. Valle-Giler EP, Sulaiman WA. Midline minimally invasive placement of spinal cord stimulators: a technical note. Ochsner J. 2014;14(1):51–6.
24. MacDonald JD, Fisher KJ. Technique for steering spinal cord stimulator electrode. Neurosurgery. 2011;69(1 Suppl Operative):ons83–6. discussion ons86-7.
25. Pabaney AH, Robin AM, Schwalb JM. New technique for open placement of paddle-type spinal cord stimulator electrode in presence of epidural scar tissue. Neuromodulation. 2014;17(8):759–62. discussion 62.
26. Robaina FJ, Dominguez M, Diaz M, Rodriguez JL, de Vera JA. Spinal cord stimulation for relief of chronic pain in vasospastic disorders of the upper limbs. Neurosurgery. 1989;24(1):63–7.
27. Amrani J. A novel technique for the implantation of paddle leads in the cervical spine. Neuromodulation. 2013;16(6):546–50. discussion 50.
28. Pahapill PA. Incidence of revision surgery in a large cohort of patients with thoracic surgical three-column paddle leads: a retrospective case review. Neuromodulation. 2015;18(5):367–75.
29. Penn DL, Zussman BM, Wu C, Sharan AD. Anterograde revision of cervical spinal cord stimulator paddle electrode: a case report. Neuromodulation. 2012;15(6):581–4. discussion 84–5.
30. Chivukula S, Tomycz ND, Moossy JJ. Paddle lead cervical spinal cord stimulation for failed neck surgery syndrome. Clin Neurol Neurosurg. 2013;115(10):2254–6.
31. Rosenow JM, Stanton-Hicks M, Rezai AR, Henderson JM. Failure modes of spinal cord stimulation hardware. J Neurosurg Spine. 2006;5(3):183–90.
32. Moens M, De Smedt A, Brouns R, Spapen H, Droogmans S, Duerinck J, et al. Retrograde C0-C1 insertion of cervical plate electrode for chronic intractable neck and arm pain. World Neurosurg. 2011;76(3–4):352–4. discussion 268–9.
33. Pahapill PA. A novel nonanchoring technique for implantation of paddle leads in the cervical spine under conscious sedation. Neuromodulation. 2015;18(6):472–6.
34. Whitworth LA, Feler CA. C1-C2 sublaminar insertion of paddle leads for the management of chronic painful conditions of the upper extremity. Neuromodulation. 2003;6(3):153–7.
35. Schu S, Slotty PJ, Bara G, von Knop M, Edgar D, Vesper J. A prospective, randomised, double-blind, placebo-controlled study to examine the effectiveness of burst spinal cord stimulation patterns for the treatment of failed back surgery syndrome. Neuromodulation. 2014;17(5):443–50.

Chapter 16
Percutaneous Placement

Konstantin V. Slavin and Dali Yin

Key Points

- Percutaneous SCS electrodes present a minimally invasive option and eliminate the need in laminectomy approach.
- Multiple advantages of percutaneous electrode leads (MRI conditional approval, ability to advance in cranio-caudal direction, ease and safety of insertion, multiple individualized configurations, etc.) should prompt neurosurgeons to become more familiar with their use.
- Spine surgery training provides an excellent background for percutaneous interventions in the epidural space.
- In a comprehensive spine surgery practice, an ability to use percutaneous SCS electrode leads widens surgeon's armamentarium and reduces dependence on outside physicians.

Introduction

Over the last 50 years or so, spinal cord stimulation (SCS) has become an established approach for management of chronic pain. As the matter of fact, it is likely the most common surgical intervention that is performed for treatment of pain both nationally and worldwide. In part, this widespread use and universal acceptance

K.V. Slavin, M.D. (✉)
Department of Neurosurgery, University of Illinois at Chicago,
912 South Wood Street, M/C 799, Rm. 451N, Chicago, IL 60612, USA
e-mail: kslavin@uic.edu

D. Yin, M.D., Ph.D.
Functional Neurosurgery, University of Illinois at Chicago, Chicago, IL USA
e-mail: daliyin@uic.edu; yindalius@yahoo.com

© Springer International Publishing Switzerland 2016
S.M. Falowski, J.E. Pope (eds.), *Integrating Pain Treatment into Your Spine Practice*, DOI 10.1007/978-3-319-27796-7_16

came from surgeons, mainly neurosurgeons, educating our nonsurgical colleagues and shifting the practice (and bulk volume) of SCS from few specialized neurosurgical centers that possessed interest, experience and expertise in surgical management of pain to myriad of pain practices, vast majority of which are run by non-surgeons.

This development became possible due to technological innovations of the early 1970s when the first cylindrical electrode leads became available. These new electrodes were a major advancement from previous flat, "plate-like" electrodes, mainly because they could be inserted into the epidural space through a needle, thereby obviating the need for open exploration to obtain access to the epidural space and, therefore, allowing non-surgeons to implant these electrode leads for trialing and permanent use.

Although earlier generations of neurosurgeons embraced percutaneously implantable electrodes, the entire premise of percutaneous access to the epidural space did not become part of standard neurosurgical armamentarium and educational curriculum. And while each neurosurgeon is expected to master craniotomies and laminectomies, training in placement of percutaneous electrodes became non-mandatory, similar to other "non-mainstream" neurosurgical skills such as stereotactic electrode insertions or endovascular interventions. There is no good explanation for this phenomenon other than lack of interest, and involvement of other specialties, as neurosurgeons are indeed very proficient with spinal needles and catheters, and routinely place lumbar drains and other intrathecal catheters as needed for diagnostic and therapeutic purposes (such as lumboperitoneal shunts, intrathecal pumps, etc.)

So, when it comes to SCS trials and implants, the spine surgeons (neurosurgeons and orthopedists specializing in spine) are expected to use flat, paddle-type, so-called surgical, or laminectomy leads—and even current educational guidelines issued by the North American Neuromodulation Society (NANS) accept neurosurgical residency as a proof of proficiency in implantation of paddle leads [1]—while use of percutaneous "wire-like" cylindrical leads is delegated to pain physicians that come from anesthesiology and physiatry backgrounds. These same NANS guidelines spell educational requirements for implantation of percutaneous electrodes in terms of volume of cases one has to perform under supervision before independent practice is allowed. This situation seemed to satisfy all parties involved (even though quite a few functional neurosurgeons continued using percutaneous implantation technique) as both percutaneous and paddle-type electrodes have their own benefits and limitations (Table 16.1).

But as technology advanced further, some limitations of percutaneous electrodes were improved upon—the high migration rate was successfully mitigated by introduction of new lockable or injectable anchors, the concern about higher energy requirements was resolved with introduction of smaller and longer-lasting batteries, as well as rechargeable devices. At the same time, new advantages of percutaneous electrodes came into play, with the most important being the MRI conditional approval of percutaneously inserted leads that opened access to SCS for many patients with oncological and demyelinating conditions that would not be considered SCS candidates earlier. In addition, new stimulation targets (such as dorsal root ganglion [DRG]) and paradigms (such as 10,000 Hz stimulation [HF10]) presently

Table 16.1 Advantages and disadvantages of different electrode types

Percutaneous leads	Paddle leads
Advantages	Advantages
Relatively lower invasiveness	Unidirectional stimulation
Relative ease of insertion	Flat contacts
Epidural insertion below the cord level	Lower power requirements
Ability to implant multiple leads at once	Insulation of dorsal tissues
Freedom to advance in cranio-caudal direction	Higher stability in epidural space
Multiple configurations possible	Fixed distance between electrode contacts
MRI compatibility (conditional)	Direct visualization of dura
Disadvantages	Disadvantages
Omnidirectional stimulation	Relatively higher invasiveness
Cylindrical contacts	Requirement of complex surgical skills
Higher power requirements	Epidural entry over the spinal cord
Lack of dorsal insulation	Challenging implantation of more than 1 lead
Higher chance of migration	Limited reach (1–2 level from laminectomy)
Variable distance between electrodes	Limited choice of configurations
Indirect visualization	Lack of full body MRI labeling

utilize percutaneous electrode leads only. At present time, the only electrode leads that are conditionally approved for MR imaging of spine (there are some MRI conditionally approved paddle leads—but only for imaging of head and extremities) are percutaneous leads. When considering this as well as the lack of paddles intended for DRG stimulation and HF10 SCS, there is now an urgent need in neurosurgeons learning or relearning to use percutaneous approach to offer their patients the newest technology in electrode leads.

Finally, there are two other recent technological innovations that should raise the level of neurosurgical interest in percutaneous lead insertion—the percutaneous paddles and wireless SCS devices. With introduction of very narrow paddle leads, it is now possible to insert one or even several of them into the epidural space without laminectomy using a proprietary percutaneous introducer system. There is also a recent introduction of miniaturized wireless spinal cord stimulation devices that contain telemetry hardware and the energy receiver in the lead itself. These devices work by coupling with an external power source and do not need implantable generator. New wireless SCS systems have been tested for MRI safety and were granted conditional approval for both 1.5 T and 3 T MRI scanners.

Temporary vs. Permanent Placement

In general, there are two reasons to implant percutaneous electrode leads. One is to use them for a short-term testing of the modality (so-called stimulation trial) and another is to provide long-term stimulation (so-called permanent implantation). Although the trial and permanent electrodes are positioned in the epidural space in a similar fashion, these interventions have their distinct nuances and may require different electrode leads as most manufacturers supply "temporary" electrode leads that are not intended for long-term stimulation and are used exclusively for trialing. The main difference between trial and permanent implantation is that trial leads are usually inserted without any incision using a pure needle-based percutaneous approach, whereas permanent implantation of percutaneous electrodes included making surgical incision and anchoring the electrode leads to the deep tissues. It is not uncommon to use percutaneous electrode leads for trial only and then to proceed with permanent implantation of paddle-type surgical electrode leads. The advantages of pure percutaneous trial is its low invasiveness, option to perform electrode lead insertion in office setting (as long as there is sterile procedure room and proper radiological control, e.g., fluoroscopy device such as C-arm), simplicity of lead removal at the end of the trial period, and lack of any incision that would require surgical skills, hemostasis, ability to suture, etc. A shortcoming of a percutaneous trial is that if the trial was successful, the lead still has to be removed and discarded, and a subsequently implanted permanent lead may need to be positioned in exactly the same location through a separate procedure (and this may be quite challenging due to development of epidural adhesions ant therefore trial results may be less predictive of long-term outcome).

In our practice, the majority of implanted SCS devices include percutaneous electrode leads—and with the use of this lead type we prefer to avoid having the patient go through electrode insertion twice. Therefore, we use the so-called "tunneled trial" approach: the trial electrode leads are inserted as if they were permanent—with incision, anchoring, etc.—and then temporary extension cables are tunneled out and used for connection to an external pulse generator (EPG). If the trial is successful, the extension cables are discarded and the electrode leads that were used for trial are kept in place and get connected to an implantable pulse generator (IPG) placed through a separate incision. The main advantage of this approach is that the same electrode lead that was used during the trial will be utilized during the permanent phase of long-term treatment thereby matching the exact location (and effects) of trial electrode placement. From a technical point of view, the lead insertion becomes easier as the skin incision and tissue dissection with visual exposure of deep fascia make accessing the epidural space less complicated and more predictable. Since the procedure is more invasive, it is usually done in a standard operating room (which is an encumbrance for non-surgeons, but a much preferred location for surgeons) with easy access to surgical instruments, fluoroscopy equipment and hemostatic tools, as well as a routinely high standard of sterility. The disadvantage of the tunneled trial technique is that if the trial fails, the patient has to return to the operating room for lead/anchor/extension cable removal. In addition, for non-surgeons, the need in proper surgical technique may be a certain deterrent.

Preparation for the Procedure

The initial steps in SCS procedure take place well in advance of the operative intervention. Proper patient selection, mandatory psychological evaluation, setting clear expectations of treatment, and detailed discussion of surgical intervention and its possible complications are key moments in the process of patient preparation for trial. The patient has to understand the concept of stimulation-induced paresthesias and be willing to participate in the trial lead insertion process as success in reaching anatomical location that produces concordant paresthesias is absolutely dependent on the patient's feedback.

It is also important to document exact anatomical location of the patient's painful areas as all of them have to be covered with non-painful paresthesias in order for SCS to be effective. Creation of so-called "pain maps" may be useful in estimation of eventual location of electrode contacts as most anatomic regions appear to have reliable correlates in terms of vertebral level of stimulation.

With this, it is important to obtain proper imaging of not only the level where the electrode will be inserted (usually, mid-lumbar or upper lumbar regions) but also the level where electrode contacts will be positioned as tight stenosis at lower thoracic levels or previous thoracic laminectomy may present significant challenge for optimal electrode lead placement.

We recommend discussing location of the generator implant with your patients beforehand—in general, our preference is to put them into the abdominal wall rather than buttock or flank area for the sake of easier recharge and programming, as well as for less discomfort during sitting and lying down. In addition, the abdominal IPG placement appears to result in less stress to the electrodes and/or extension cables thereby reducing the risk of migration or fracture [2]. The side of IPG implantation is dictated by patient's individual anatomy, presence of surgical scars, shunts, stomas or external tubes, as well as by the patient's driving status as those who drive may want to have the IPG on the left side of the abdomen so it does not interfere with the seatbelt position whereas for those spending more time in the passenger seat the opposite may be true.

The last concerns to be addressed prior to the lead insertion are the planned position of the active lead contacts, estimated number of leads (1–4) and contacts per lead (4–16), and the type of electrode lead to be used (manufacturer and model), including the number of contacts, length of the lead and the need in anchors and extension cables as this information has to be communicated with the vendor who will have requested devices available along with the mandatory backup devices in case of intraoperative technical challenges.

Procedural Detail

The procedure starts from positioning the patient prone on a radiolucent table (Fig. 16.1). C-arm fluoroscopy device is placed around the patient to obtain antero-posterior view of the thoracolumbar junction and the upper lumbar spine (Fig. 16.2) as most electrode leads have to be positioned at the low thoracic level. The area of intervention is prepped and draped in a standard sterile fashion—the size of surgical field is determined by whether there is a plan to anchor the electrode lead(s) and tunnel the extension cables or if the lead(s) will be simply inserted for trial purposes only; tunneling necessitates wider area of preparation (Fig. 16.3). Based on the

Fig. 16.1 Patient
positioned prone on the
operating table

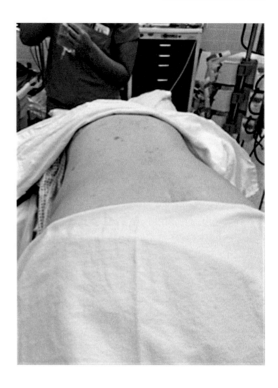

Fig. 16.2 C-arm
fluoroscopy device is
positioned around the
patient

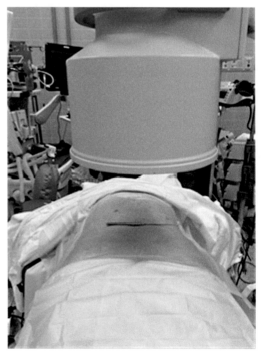

Fig. 16.3 Levels of
surgery are marked on the
patient's skin

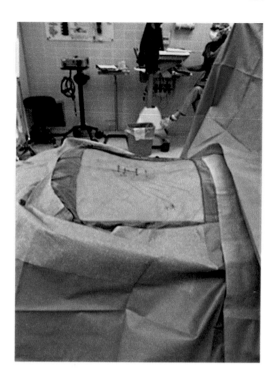

planned location of IPG, it is recommended to tunnel temporary extension cables in the opposite direction, so that the exit site of the temporary extensions does not get on the way of eventual tunneling path toward IPG. This is also important in decreasing risk of an infection from the previous externalized extensions.

The entry into epidural space is usually chosen at L1-2 or L2-3 interspace level. In general, it is recommended to place the needle entry below the level of the spinal cord conus in order to minimize the risk of spinal cord injury during needle and electrode lead insertion. From this upper lumbar insertion level it is possible to place SCS lead(s) anywhere along the spinal cord all the way to C2, but for cervical lead placement we prefer using high thoracic epidural entry point that is much more technically challenging and is not recommended for those with limited experience.

Although most electrodes are positioned over the midline, the needle insertion point has to be paramedian, at least 1 or 2 cm away from the midline. This paramedian insertion allows one to avoid positioning the electrode lead between the spinous processes. This position may lead to repetitive compression of the implanted lead by the bone and would inevitably result in lead fracture. Usually, a 30° angle in axial plane would suffice for paramedian direction of the needle (Fig. 16.4). Similarly, the needle has to be obliquely directed in cranio-caudal plane: perpendicular needle insertion (at 90° angle to the skin surface) results in more challenging identification of the epidural space and significant difficulty in advancing the lead out of the needle tip inside the epidural space. Usually, a 30°–45° angle is chosen.

Fig. 16.4 Insertion of
needle into epidural space

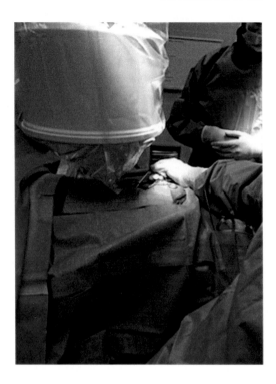

The needle used for electrode lead insertion is a special Tuohy-type needle that is provided in the electrode lead kit from every manufacturer. Most kits would include a 4 in. long needle with a marching stylet; longer needles (6 in.) are available upon request. These needles have a sharp tip and a side opening to facilitate penetration of soft tissues, including ligamentum flavum, but make it easier to direct the exiting electrode lead into the epidural space with the use of this bevel. There are also "Coude-type" needles with a more curved tip; we do not recommend using them for antegrade electrode insertions.

For pure temporary percutaneous electrode lead insertion (non-tunneled), the skin entry point is usually chosen one and a half vertebral levels below the interspace chosen for epidural entry. Laterality of such entry correlates with location of the vertebral pedicle. Therefore, for L2-L3 epidural entry, the skin entry marked over projection of pedicle of L4; for L1-L2—pedicle of L3. For insertion of two electrodes, the entry points are chosen on both sides of the same level or on two levels on the same side. Alternatively, for percutaneous electrode leads intended for tunneled trial, the midline incision is usually made in the same fashion—at the level of L3-L4 for L1-L2 insertion and at the level of L4-L5 for L2-L3 insertion. In this case, the incision is made in vertical direction, 2–4 cm in length depending on the patient's size, and the fascia is exposed on both sides of midline. We recommend creating a small pocket above the fascia under the subcutaneous adipose layer in order to make room for anchors, electrode loops and connectors to temporary extension cables. Making this pocket prior to insertion of the leads eliminates the need for tissue manipulation after the electrode leads are in place and reduces the risk of inadvertent lead damage during tissue dissection or migration after placement. The size of subcutaneous pocket should be 2–3 cm wide and 2–4 cm long. It is also recommended to insert the needle into the fascia in the most superior aspect of the exposed fascia to there is room for anchors caudal to the insertion point. Inserting the needle in the middle of the incision or more caudal would usually necessitate caudal extension of the skin incision.

The needle is directed toward the midline from paramedian entry point. The anatomy of the epidural space is such that the space is thickest over the midline— the somewhat triangular shape of spinal canal with apex at midline is not perfectly matched by the oval shape of thecal sac. The midline epidural space is usually 2–4 mm thick, but there is individual variability, as well as possible presence of stenosis and/or scar tissue from previous interventions may make the space narrower. The posterior epidural space is filled with fat and vessels. The softness of epidural fat contrasts with the hardness of ligaments that define epidural space dorsally; this difference in density translates into so-called "loss of resistance" phenomenon. An experienced implanter would feel entry into the epidural space based on tactile feedback, particularly with proper radiographic guidance, but is generally recommended to confirm this loss of resistance by gentle injection of saline or air during the needle advancement. For this, the needle is inserted with the stylet in and the interosseous space is gently probed. Once the interlaminar space if entered, the stylet is removed and a plastic or glass syringe is attached to the needle hub. As the advancement continues, a gentle pressure is applied to the syringe plunger; once the epidural space is entered, the resistance of tissues disappears and the syringe ~1 ml of contents (be that air or saline) gets injected into the epidural space. At this point, it is recommended to disengage the syringe and confirm that there is no fluid flowing from the needle hub to make sure that the needle did not go too deep and inadvertently penetrate the dura.

We routinely use a guidewire that comes in the lead insertion kit for testing the loss of resistance: instead of syringe with air or saline, we insert this guidewire into the Tuohy needle after the needle tip passes between the laminae and enters the ligamentum flavum. As soon as the needle penetrates the ligament, the guidewire is advanced into the epidural space under fluoroscopic control. As the guidewire pushes away the underlying dura, it becomes easier and safer to advance the needle by another millimeter or two allowing positioning of the entire needle tip opening into the epidural space. This minor needle advancement facilitates subsequent insertion of the electrode lead into the epidural space.

Once the needle is positioned in the epidural space (Fig. 16.5), we recommend a short run of live fluoroscopy during initial part of electrode lead insertion as the angle at which it leaves the needle is crucial for ultimate lead positioning. Here, the lead should be placed as close to the midline as possible since lateral deviation of the lead may result in its circling around the thecal sac and getting into the ventral epidural space instead of remaining in the posterior epidural space. If the plan is to insert a single lead, we prefer placing it at midline with only mild deviation toward the side of worse pain. If two electrodes are contemplated, each would be placed

Fig. 16.5 Fluoroscopic image of paramedian needle insertion

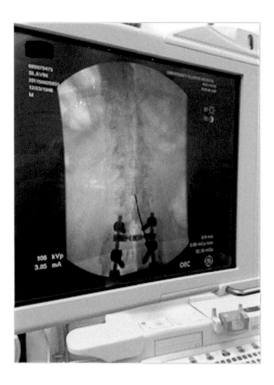

next to midline for patients with bilateral pain or one would be placed at midline and another 2–3 mm lateral toward the side of pain in patients with unilateral pain. Use of curved stylets that are provided in the lead kits and are frequently preloaded into the leads facilitates easy steering of the lead during its epidural advancement (Fig. 16.6).

The level of electrode contacts is determined by the patient's pain location and adjusted based on results of intraoperative stimulation. During intraoperative testing, the electrode leads are connected to a sterile single-use screening cable (Fig. 16.7) which then connects to an external (non-sterile) programmer that is held outside of the sterile field by a dedicated assistant or clinical specialist from the device manufacturer. The patient sedation is stopped prior to initiation of intraoperative testing. Since it is easier to pull electrode out rather than advance it in further during the intraoperative testing stage, we prefer to intentionally advance the lead higher than needed and then, during the testing, "trawl" it down until desired coverage is obtained. We recommend removing the stylet from each electrode lead prior to starting the intraoperative testing.

The patient is usually asked three questions: when paresthesia starts, where it is felt, and whether all painful areas are properly covered. We do not ask the patients whether stimulation reduces or eliminates their pain as it may take several hours or even days of stimulation before the pain relief becomes noticeable. In addition, it may be difficult for the patient to discern pain relief while on the operating table. Ideally the paresthesias should be completely concordant with spreading into all painful areas with minimal involvement of non-painful regions. Proper coverage of

Fig. 16.6 Fluoroscopic
view of percutaneous
electrode lead being
advanced in cephalad
direction

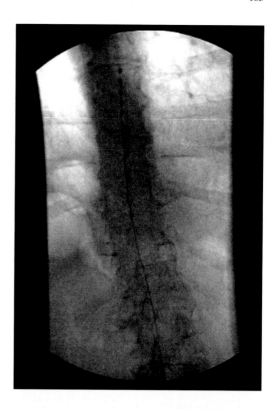

Fig. 16.7 Electrode tails
are connected to the
screening cable for
intraoperative stimulation
trial

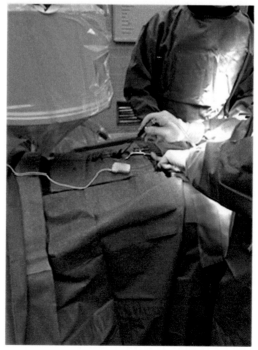

painful areas is of paramount importance in conventional spinal cord stimulation as some patients will not get good pain relief even if paresthesias are concordant, but no patient will get pain relief if paresthesias do not match the area of pain. Sometimes, the best stimulation may shift by contact or two after the patient changes position from prone to supine. To be prepared for this contingency, we recommend trying to get best stimulation from the middle of the electrode array, aiming to place the middle of the lead on what has become known as "the sweet spot". Given this positioning of the lead, even if the spinal cord moves relative to the electrode lead after position change, the proper stimulation coverage may still be obtained using adjacent electrode contacts.

The implanters should be aware that not only may individual dermatomal distribution vary from person to person, but that radiographic midline may be very different from physiological midline. In addition, this difference is even more pronounced in patients with scoliosis. With this, it is not uncommon to position two electrodes side by side on both sides of radiographic midline and then discover that patient feels stimulation from both leads on the same side. In such cases, the more lateral electrode has to be pulled down and readvanced on the opposite side of the other electrode.

Only after paresthesias are mapped and confirmed, can the needles be removed. The electrode lead position gets recorded with intraoperative fluoroscopy and the image (with proper landmarks such as, for example, 12th ribs) gets saved on the screen for subsequent comparison. After the needles are removed, the electrode leads get anchored to the fascia (or to the skin in case of temporary trials). The anchor is placed as close to the fascia as possible (Fig. 16.8); most anchor models have a narrow "nozzle" that may be inserted into the fascia prior to the anchor suturing. The sutures used for anchoring are 2-0 non-absorbable braided dacron (Ethibond or Surgi-Dac) or silk (Fig. 16.9). We do not recommend using either absorbable (Vicryl, Polysorb) or monofilament (Prolene, Monocryl) sutures for this purpose.

Once the anchoring is completed, a control radiograph is obtained and compared with pre-anchoring image. After that, we proceed with tunneling the temporary extension cables to an exit point 10–12 cm away from the midline (Fig. 16.10) and then connect these cables to each electrode lead. Once the connection is secured with set screws, the excess of the electrode leads and the connectors are buried under the skin, the incision gets irrigated with antibiotic solution, the hemostasis is obtained with bipolar coagulation (use of monopolar stimulation after the electrode is inserted into the epidural space is not recommended), and the closure is performed in layers. The dressing is placed over the incision and over the exit site of the extension cables (Fig. 16.11). The impedance of electrode contacts is tested by connecting the extensions to the screening cable and running diagnostic testing through the external programmer.

Fig. 16.8 Electrodes are
anchored to the fascia

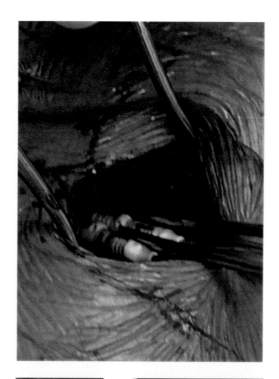

Fig. 16.9 Two
nonabsorbable sutures are
placed over each anchor,
which is fixed onto the
fascia

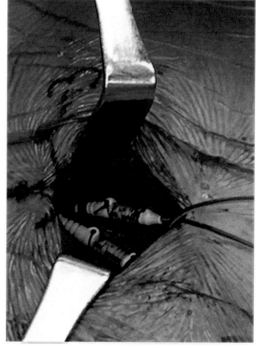

Fig. 16.10 Tunneling for extension cables, and connection between electrodes and extension cables

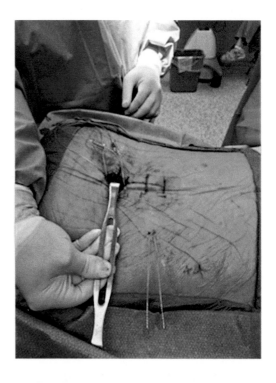

Fig. 16.11 Sterile dressings over the incision and the exit site of the extension cables

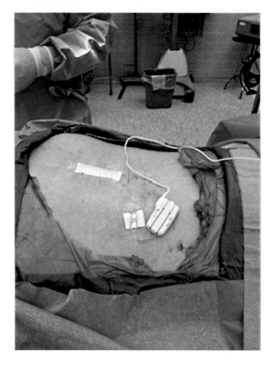

Summary

Proper electrode insertion is one of the most important technical parts of the spinal cord stimulation approach, but it translates into a good outcome only if other aspects are addressed with similarly meticulous attention to detail. This includes patient selection, trialing process, permanent implantation procedure, and subsequent patient management, all of which are discussed in other parts of this book. Percutaneous technique is remarkably simple and intuitive for those who are familiar with spinal anatomy and are willing to spend time and effort in practicing the approach on several occasions. Although an alternative technique of using surgical paddle leads attracts spinal surgeons from neurosurgical and orthopedic backgrounds, recent introduction of new features, targets and paradigms that are only available with percutaneous lead options (full body MRI-conditional compatibility, high frequency stimulation, dorsal root ganglion stimulation, etc.) should prompt them to learn percutaneous technique in order to continue providing their patients with the best treatment options.

References

1. Henderson JM, Levy RM, Bedder MD, Staats PS, Slavin KV, Poree LR, North RB. NANS training requirements for spinal cord stimulation devices: selection, implantation, and follow-up. Neuromodulation. 2009;12:171–4.
2. Henderson JM, Schade CM, Sasaki J, Caraway D, Oakley J. Prevention of mechanical failures in implanted spinal cord stimulation systems. Neuromodulation. 2006;9:183–91.

Chapter 17
Peripheral Nerve Stimulation—Cervical Syndromes

Joshua M. Rosenow

Key Points

- Peripheral stimulation may be utilized to treat a variety of cervical pain syndromes, either localized pain or pain referred from upper cervical root neuralgias.
- The published series on these techniques show good rates of conversion of trials to permanent implants.
- The published series on these techniques are mostly small retrospective series, which limits their generalizability.
- These procedures are straightforward and relatively simple to perform.
- Device-related complications such as lead migration remain the most significant long term issue with these procedures. Adherence to good surgical techniques can minimize these problems.

Introduction

Neurostimulation is an attractive technique for the treatment of medically refractory pain syndromes. Minimally invasive implantation of neurostimulation electrodes often provides significant pain relief via a reversible and adjustable therapy with low medical and surgical risks. While neurostimulation is most often employed for treatment of axial and radicular lumbar syndromes, cervical pain syndromes are

J.M. Rosenow, M.D., F.A.A.N.S., F.A.C.S. (✉)
Departments of Neurosurgery, Neurology and Physical Medicine and Rehabilitation,
Northwestern University Feinberg School of Medicine,
676 N. St. Clair St., Suite 2210, Chicago, IL 60611, USA
e-mail: JRosenow@nm.org

© Springer International Publishing Switzerland 2016   191
S.M. Falowski, J.E. Pope (eds.), *Integrating Pain Treatment into Your Spine Practice*, DOI 10.1007/978-3-319-27796-7_17

being treated with increasing frequency. This is being driven in large part due to improvements in neurostimulation device technology. Advances such as 8- and 16-contact percutaneous electrodes, slender 8-contact paddle electrodes, ultrasound guidance, and programming options such as a wider parameter space and current steering, all enable physicians to treat a wider range of pain conditions.

This chapter discusses the use of peripheral stimulation for the treatment of cervical syndromes such as axial cervical pain, cervicogenic headache, and occipital neuralgia.

Evidence

Unfortunately the body of scientific evidence for these procedures is rather sparse. Recently, an excellent evidence-based guidelines document has been published that analyzed the literature on the use of peripheral (occipital) nerve stimulation for the treatment of refractory occipital neuralgia (C2 neuralgia) [1]. No articles have been better than class III evidence. The large prospective series is that of Melvin et al. [2] and consisted of only 16 patients, 11 of which underwent a successful trial of stimulation and proceeded to permanent implantation. In these patients there was a statistically significant decline in SF-MPQ (64 % change, $p = 0.0013$), VAS (67 % change, $p < 0.0001$), and PPI (67 % change, $p = 0.0009$) at 12 weeks following permanent system implantation. Smaller series by Magown et al. [3] and Kapural et al. [4] demonstrated similar improvements in pain levels, as well as improvements in standardized scales such as the Pain Disability Index (PDI).

Retrospective series are only slightly larger. Weiner and Reed's seminal series [5] included 13 patients, all of whom continued to report greater than 50 % pain relief at a mean follow-up of 2 years. In the series of Slavin et al. [6], 10 of 14 patients underwent successful trials, with three systems removed during the mean of 22 months follow-up. The 7 remaining patients continued report greater than 60 % pain relief at last follow-up.

There are no randomized trials investigating the choice of stimulating lead (percutaneous vs. paddle lead). Series by Abhinav [7], Magown [3], Oh [8], and Kapural [4] all documented successful use of subcutaneously placed paddle electrodes.

Migration is one of the more common complications of these procedures and the series of Slavin et al. [6] (10 patients, percutaneous electrodes) and Oh et al. [8] (10 patients, paddle electrodes) both reported a 10 % migration rate. However, in larger series of patients who underwent occipital stimulation for treatment of primary cranial pain the reported migration rate was between 13.9 and 24 %. Falowski et al. reported on a series of 28 patients demonstrating a significant decrease in the rate of migration utilizing specific anchoring techniques and strain relief loops [9].

The reported series of patients who underwent trials and neurostimulation device implantation for regional cervical pain are also small. Burgher's et al. series [10] only contained 1 of 10 patients with cervical pain, as opposed to lumbar pain. Lipov [11] reported a single case of regional stimulation for axial cervical pain.

Implementation

In planning a peripheral neurostimulation system for a specific patient, several factors need to be considered. First and foremost is the target structure to be stimulated. This is dictated by the region of pain and consideration needs to be given to whether the target is a named nerve or a geographic region. The type of lead to be implanted (paddle, percutaneous) needs to be decided. Next, the placement of the pulse generator needs to be discussed with the patient, as this may also dictate the surgical approach for lead placement. Often, these factors are interrelated and their competing priorities decide the overall implant approach.

Cervical peripheral stimulation trials are almost always performed using percutaneously inserted electrodes. If the stimulation target is a named nerve (such as the greater or lesser occipital nerve), the path of the electrode should be planned in close relationship to the path of the nerve. In many cases, this results in perpendicular orientation as the electrode crosses the path of the nerve. However, the electrode can also be placed parallel to the nerve, especially if ultrasound guidance is successful at identifying the nerve.

In placing the trial electrodes, standard stainless steel Touhy needles (such as those included in most spinal cord stimulation electrode lead kits) may be used. These should be appropriately curved to approximate the patient's anatomy. The bevel of the needle should be pointed away from the skin surface to reduce the chance of violating the skin. Usually only a small stab incision is needed for insertion. The proper plane is located just beneath the dermis and not too deep so as to cause muscular contractions. However, in patients with very thick subcutaneous fat, it may be necessary to place the electrode deeper so as to facilitate the current reaching the target structure. After confirmation of paresthesia coverage the lead may be sutured to the skin for the duration of the trial.

If performing stimulation for regional pain, a box demarcating the area of pain should be marked off on the skin. The insertion needles and electrodes can then be inserted subcutaneously along the borders of this box to bracket the painful region (Fig. 17.1). Stimulation may be conducted either with the electrodes being used independently or via a stimulation field set up between the electrodes.

For a stimulation trial, the electrodes may be stabilized by suturing them to the skin with a combination purse-string/drain suture. However, for a permanent stimulation system implantation, anchoring the electrodes is one of the more crucial steps, as electrode migration is one of the most frequently reported complications of these procedures. When anchoring the leads, it is important to identify a firm stable tissue layer to which to anchor the leads. In the cervical region this is often the most superficial layer of posterior cervical fascia. Anchoring to subcutaneous fat layers often leads to an unstable electrode that migrates with cervical motion. It should be noted that the anchoring depth is often deeper than the insertion depth. Given this, it is reasonable to first dissect down to the anchoring layer and then insert the needle and electrode more superficially during a permanent implant procedure.

Fig. 17.1 Example of regional peripheral stimulation (in this case for axial thoracic pain). The two sets of electrodes have been inserted subcutaneously along the length of the demarcated lateral borders of the patient's painful region. Successful stimulation coverage for this patient was achieved via a combination of programs that used both the electrodes independently and in cross-talk configuration

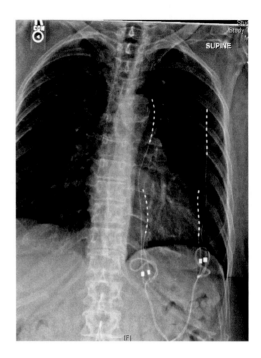

Electrodes may be anchored with commercially available anchoring sleeves. If these are used, efforts should be made to avoid having the entire anchor located underneath the incision, so as to reduce the chance of erosion. The least bulky anchor possible should be utilized. Some physicians have chosen to forgo a formal anchor sleeve altogether and simply suture the lead to the fascia. It remains to be seen if this increases the chance of electrode fatigue and breakage over time. Subcutaneous pockets are may also be created around the main incision for placement of relaxing electrode loops to add slack to the system.

For permanent implantation, either percutaneous of paddle electrodes may be used. Percutaneous electrodes are now available in multiple configurations with anywhere from 4 to 16 stimulating contacts on the electrode. Electrodes with 16 contacts may enable the capture of bilateral greater occipital nerves with a single lead. To place a subcutaneous paddle lead a pocket for the body of the paddle must be created. This is typically done with gentle blunt dissection. It is important not to be overly aggressive and make this pocket much larger than the paddle body. Doing so not only can increase the diffusion of charge away from the target structure but also leads to more mobility of the electrode, which is suboptimal both in terms of comfort (patients feel the paddle rotating) and consistency of therapy.

When implanting upper cervical peripheral stimulating electrodes (those intended to treat syndromes such as cervicogenic headache and occipital neuralgia), several incision configurations may be used. If bilateral leads are to be tunneled to a generator implanted in the infraclavicular region, two incisions may be used: a submastoid incision ipsilateral to the generator and a midline incision (Fig. 17.2). For generators implanted in other dorsal locations, a single midline incision may be created with the electrodes both anchored in the same incision (Fig. 17.3).

Fig. 17.2 Percutaneously
implanted upper cervical
electrodes for stimulation
of the occipital nerves.
These were implanted via
two separate incisions, one
in the submastoid region
and another in the midline

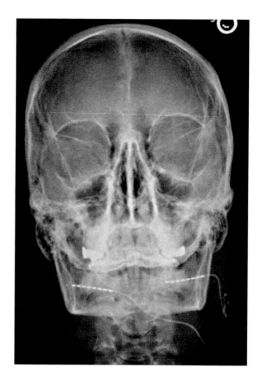

Fig. 17.3 Percutaneously
implanted upper cervical
electrodes for stimulation
of the occipital nerves.
These were implanted via a
single midline incision.
Note the relaxing loops
present caudal to the
electrodes

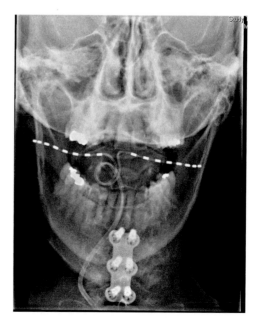

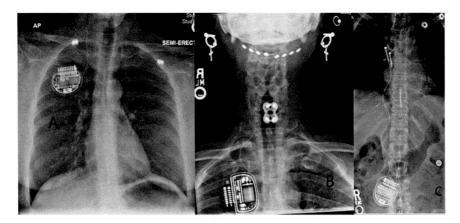

Fig. 17.4 Examples of locations for peripheral stimulation IPG sites. (**a**) Infraclavicular region, (**b**) midline dorsal upper thoracic (note paddle electrodes used in this case), (**c**) lumbar (note extension wires added in upper thoracic region to increase slack in the system and reduce risk of electrode migration)

When performing peripheral stimulation procedures in the cervical region, there are several options for locating the implantable pulse generator (IPG) (Fig. 17.4). The leads may be tunneled laterally and over the clavicle to an IPG implanted in the upper chest. This provides for a short electrode distance (often without the need for extension wires) but may place torque on the leads with cervical motion, increasing the chance of lead migration if they are not securely anchored. The IPG may also be placed in the midline interscapular region. This allows for a shorter lead length with less force on the lead. If this location is considered, the patient should be observed sitting in chairs with backs of various heights to ensure that the IPG will not cause discomfort when the patient sits back against the chair. Another option is to place the IPG in the low back/upper buttock region. This will require the longest length of lead and often also requires the use of an extension wire down to the IPG site. For IPG implants in this location, attention must be paid to the total length of implanted lead/extension so that there is enough slack in the system to allow significant range of motion in both the cervical and lumbar regions without pulling the electrodes.

For many peripheral nerve stimulation procedures in the cervical region, no image guidance is required. Fluoroscopy can be a valuable adjunct in occipital nerve stimulator electrode implants because the level of the ring of C1 is often used as a marker to help establish the craniocaudal position of these electrodes. Ultrasound may be used instead of fluoroscopy. This allows real time visualization of the relationship between the implant needle/electrode and the nerve and major vasculature without exposing the physician to ionizing radiation.

Summary

Peripheral nerve stimulation is a relatively straightforward technique for the treatment of cervical pain syndromes. Adherence to good surgical practices is important to reduce device-related complications. While this method is increasingly employed, the available scientific evidence is plagued by methodological flaws and small sample sizes.

References

1. Sweet JA, Mitchell LS, Narouze S, Sharan AD, Falowski SM, Schwalb JM, et al. Occipital nerve stimulation for the treatment of patients with medically refractory occipital neuralgia: congress of neurological surgeons systematic review and evidence-based guideline. Neurosurgery. 2015;77(3):332–41. PubMed.
2. Melvin Jr EA, Jordan FR, Weiner RL, Primm D. Using peripheral stimulation to reduce the pain of C2-mediated occipital headaches: a preliminary report. Pain Physician. 2007;10(3):453–60. PubMed.
3. Magown P, Garcia R, Beauprie I, Mendez IM. Occipital nerve stimulation for intractable occipital neuralgia: an open surgical technique. Clin Neurosurg. 2009;56:119–24. PubMed.
4. Kapural L, Mekhail N, Hayek SM, Stanton-Hicks M, Malak O. Occipital nerve electrical stimulation via the midline approach and subcutaneous surgical leads for treatment of severe occipital neuralgia: a pilot study. Anesth Analg. 2005;101(1):171–4, table of contents. PubMed.
5. Weiner RL, Reed KL. Peripheral neurostimulation for control of intractable occipital neuralgia. Neuromodulation. 1999;2(3):217–21. PubMed.
6. Slavin KV, Nersesyan H, Wess C. Peripheral neurostimulation for treatment of intractable occipital neuralgia. Neurosurgery. 2006;58(1):112–9. discussion 112–9. PubMed.
7. Abhinav K, Park ND, Prakash SK, Love-Jones S, Patel NK. Novel use of narrow paddle electrodes for occipital nerve stimulation—technical note. Neuromodulation. 2013;16(6):607–9. PubMed.
8. Oh MY, Ortega J, Bellotte JB, Whiting DM, Alo K. Peripheral nerve stimulation for the treatment of occipital neuralgia and transformed migraine using a c1-2-3 subcutaneous paddle style electrode: a technical report. Neuromodulation. 2004;7(2):103–12. PubMed.
9. Falowski S, Wang D, Sabesan A, Sharan A. Occipital nerve stimulator systems: review of complications and surgical techniques. Neuromodulation. 2010;13(2):121–5.
10. Burgher AH, Huntoon MA, Turley TW, Doust MW, Stearns LJ. Subcutaneous peripheral nerve stimulation with inter-lead stimulation for axial neck and low back pain: case series and review of the literature. Neuromodulation. 2012;15(2):100–6. discussion 6–7. PubMed.
11. Lipov EG, Joshi JR, Sanders S, Slavin KV. Use of peripheral subcutaneous field stimulation for the treatment of axial neck pain: a case report. Neuromodulation. 2009;12(4):292–5. PubMed.

Chapter 18
Peripheral Nerve Stimulation for Axial Pain Syndromes

W. Porter McRoberts

Key Points

- Axial pain is difficult to treat both surgically and nonsurgically. Traditional spinal cord stimulation (SCS) has great difficulty generating paresthesia as well as pain relief in these areas.
- The morphology of the spinal cord and entering nerves predispose electrical recruitment of the sensory fibers of the extremities long before activation of the axial sensory nerves.
- Peripheral nerve field stimulation (PNfS) is described as the blind deployment of electrodes in the subcutaneous periphery deep to the skin over unnamed nerves.
- Cross talk and hybrid stimulation force the conduction of electricity via a circuit between electrodes distant from each other, and thus large areas of paresthesia are generated.
- PNfS is currently off-label for most traditional neuromodulation systems.
- Newer waveforms and current densities may have increased ability to treat axial pain syndromes, but at present little data exists to suggest successful low back pain treatment, and far less exists to recommend treatment of the painful axial thoracic or cervical spinal areas.

W.P. McRoberts, M.D. (✉)
Interventional Spine and Pain Medicine, Neurosurgery, Holy Cross Hospital,
3111 NE 44th St., Ft. Lauderdale, FL 33308, USA
e-mail: portermcroberts@gmail.com

© Springer International Publishing Switzerland 2016
S.M. Falowski, J.E. Pope (eds.), *Integrating Pain Treatment into Your Spine Practice*, DOI 10.1007/978-3-319-27796-7_18

Introduction

Any surgeon reading this text knows that axial spinal pain is a "bear to treat." What follows is a description of the methodology and rationale for an effective but controversial method for treating axial pain with neuromodulation, peripheral nerve field stimulation. PNfS was likely initially developed simultaneously by both Giancarlo Barolat [1] and Teo Goroszeniuk [2] in the early 2000s. The aim was to provide paresthetic coverage of difficult-to-treat areas such as the axial areas overlying the low back, thoracic spine, as well as the neck. There exists no optimal treatment for pain syndromes in these axial areas of yet. Traditional SCS, when placed over the dorsal columns, excels at treatment of radicular, buttock, and neuropathic pain, but for several neurophysiologic reasons largely fails at treatment of axial pain [3]. The more central and more cephalad the pain exists, the more difficult it is to treat [4–6].

The topographic arrangement of the axial target neurons, those second-order sensory neurons in the dorsal columns which serve sensation to the spine and back, projects rostrally in the most lateral tracts (Fig. 18.1) [7]. Additionally, these axial sensory projections are generally of small fiber type, which neurophysiologically are activated at stimulation thresholds many orders lower than larger fibers. Adjacent to these lateral tracts are several sets of large fibers, which are either useless to the modulation of pain or painful to stimulate. Large, dorsal spinocerebellar tract fibers run nearby and are also likely to be activated by SCS [8, 9]. Lastly, the maximum stimulus allowed in SCS exceeds perception threshold by only 40 % and compounding difficulty, the maximum depth that fibers within the cord can be

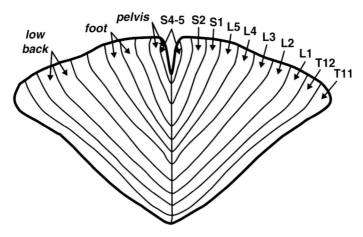

Fig. 18.1 The somatotopic organization of the thoracic dorsal columns: Note the proximity of the low back fibers to the lateral portions of the column and thus the entering dorsal root entry zone fibers from the thoracic rootlets. From Holsheimer J. Does dual lead stimulation favor stimulation of the axial lower back? Neuromodulation 2000;3(2):55–7. Reprinted with permission from Jan Holsheimer and John Wiley and Sons

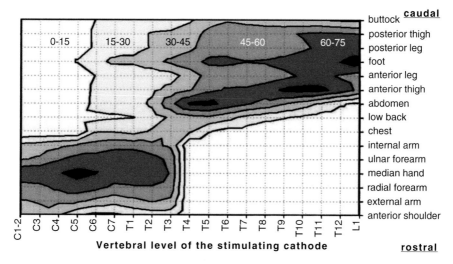

Fig. 18.2 A three-dimensional plot showing the probability of paresthesia contours as a function of the vertebral level of epidural stimulation. From Holsheimer J, Barolat G. Spinal geometry and paresthesia coverage in spinal cord stimulation. Neuromodulation, 1998;1(3):129–36. Reprinted with permission from Jan Holsheimer and John Wiley and Sons

activated is about 0.2–0.25 mm [8]. There is simply a small paresthetic window for low back and axial coverage because long before stimulation of the target fibers occurs—painful stimulation of nearby DREZ and other fibers occurs (Fig. 18.2) [10]. The physiologic problem becomes compounded as one moves cephalad. In short, searching for the low back fibers in the cord parallels the proverbial needle search in the haystack. This challenge has been the impetus for development of tripolar as well as multicolumn arrays, which while improving the chances of axial coverage still have great difficulty of providing lasting relief.

Practice and Technique of PNfS and Hybrid Stimulation (HS) in the Axial Space

From the neurophysiological frustrations described above arose PNfS and HS. PNfS enjoys as its almost sole audience the subcutaneous sensory fibers, which synapse at the dorsal horn. In the majority of cases, there exist no other electrically active neural fibers nearby. There exist three separate approaches to stimulation of the axial back and neck: (1) direct peripheral nerve stimulation, which is stimulation of a target nerve, such as the cluneal or thoracic intercostal nerves for stimulation of pain within that neural watershed; (2) PNfS which is defined as stimulation of the subcutaneous tissues by placing an electrode array wholly under the skin in the area of pain within the local watershed; and (3) hybrid stimulation defined as cross-talking electrical stimulation from electrodes at a distance from each other, be it electrical circuit from periphery to periphery [11], or between the spinal cord and the periphery. The use of PNfS and HS is based on the concept that the delivery of current to a specific peripheral nerve or DRG will affect transmission of pain influencing the firing of the A-delta and C fibers, as well as possibly change the neurotransmitters in the tissue. Although the exact mechanism of PNfS is unknown, it is thought to rely on the "gate-control theory" put forth by Melzack and Wall [12]. This theory proposed that the activation of low-threshold myelinated primary afferent fibers decreases the response of dorsal horn neurons to unmyelinated nociceptors through competitive inhibition.

The placement of a PNfS lead, while appearing easy, is dependent on the area of target pain. Pain outside the area of paresthesia will not be influenced, so the aim is to produce a net of depolarizing current, which will serve to depolarize the A-beta fibers and competitively inhibit A-delta and C fibers at the dorsal horn. Electrodes should be placed to frame the painful area, casting the net either within the periphery itself or between the spinal canal/cord and the periphery. Having the patient mark the painful areas on the skin is additionally very helpful, especially if done over the days preceding the trial (see Figs. 18.4 and 18.6).

Flank pain following spinal fusion might be trialed as seen in Fig. 18.3, one lead overlying the spinal cord, one lead in the gutter, overlying the post-ganglionic afferent dorsal root entry zone fibers, one PNfS lead superior to the painful area, and one inferior, one anterior. The trial patient seen in Fig. 18.3 was implanted with two leads in the canal and two in the periphery, one posteriorly, one anteriorly.

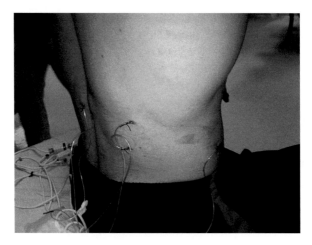

Fig. 18.3 A photo showing multiple central and peripheral leads. From the left to right: An SCS lead over the right dorsal column, an SCS lead covering the right T12–L1 dorsal root entry zone fibers, two thoracic intercostal nerve peripheral nerve stimulation leads, and lastly in the anterior a PNfS lead cross-talked to the central leads

Fig. 18.4 A
dermatographic
representation of the pain
and its intensity with lead
locations noted in barred
areas

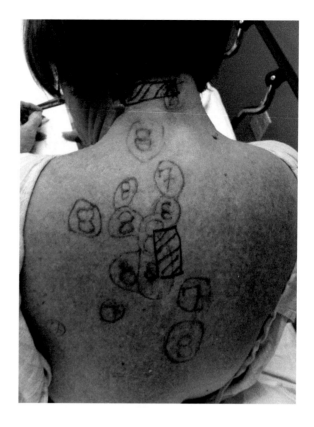

Posterior, high axial cervical and complex thoracic pain following attempted keyhole and cervical laminoplasty might be trialed in the following manner: SCS lead over the posterior dorsal columns in the low cervical region, and then one lead superficially just near the area of maximal pain in cervical area and a second lead in the area of maximal pain in thoracic spine, as can be seen in Figs. 18.4 and 18.5. Since the density of paresthesia is divisible by the area stimulated, the decision to sacrifice the right, low thoracic midline 7-8/10 pain was made to likely capture the midthoracic pain seen surrounding the lead placement there. Additionally, as can be seen in Fig. 18.4, asking the patient to make a dermatographic representation of the existing pain aids planning of lead placement significantly (Fig. 18.6).

Focal, axial spinal pain, perhaps the most demanding to treat with SCS alone, is often well treated with SCS leads in conjunction with overlying PNfS leads, forming an HS field of paresthesia programmed to place either cathode or anode in the canal with the corresponding electrode in the periphery overlying the pain (see Figs. 18.7, 18.8, and 18.9). Interestingly, it has been the observation of the authors and others that with HS programming, even if one anesthetizes the skin and periphery with local anesthetic around the peripherally placed lead, one can still cross-talk program to obtain principally axial paresthesia—indicating that neither the peripheral

Fig. 18.5 The radiographic representation of the planned patient noted in Fig. 18.4

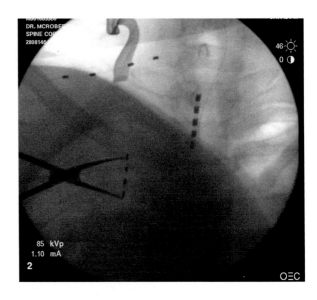

Fig. 18.6 Pain mapping the thoracic spine after fusion from high cervical to low lumbar spine

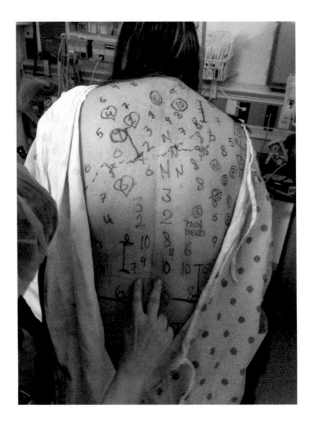

Fig. 18.7 Programming of overlying leads and cross talk between SCS and PNfS

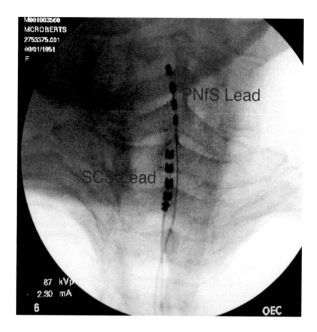

Fig. 18.8 Programming of left thoracic posterior wall pain with cross talk

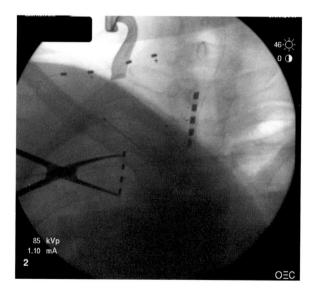

cutaneous nerves nor the ascending dorsal sensory tracts are likely the primarily depolarized neural tissue, as the peripheral nerves are chemically impeded and the dorsal tracts represent primarily radicular projections to areas where patients do not typically report paresthesia. They rather report axial paresthesia—indicating depolarization of either DREZ, DRG, or large, axial peripheral nerves.

Fig. 18.9 Programming of very focal thoracic pain with overlying PNfS lead in the horizontal position

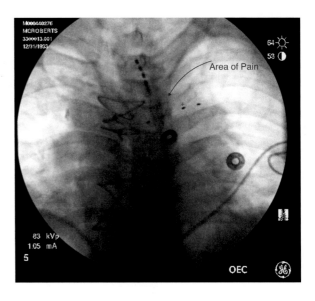

Evidence

PNS is neither new nor experimental. PNS was the first tested and reported invasive neuromodulatory device used to treat pain in 1967 when Wall and Sweet published their sentinel, "Temporary abolition of pain in man" [13]. Since that time, significant case studies have demonstrated effect and technique, but to date PNS and PNfS lack the scientific effort seen to substantiate SCS. Several case series have suggested PNfS as effective for truncal pain. Paicus et al. [14] first reported a case series of six patients, five of whom had undergone previous surgery, and all noting at least 50 % pain relief. Verrills et al. [15] reported a consecutive case series of patients with PNfS in which 85 % reported at least 50 % pain relief. Discographically confirmed cervical discogenic pain was treated with 100 % improvement with PNfS at 9-month follow-up [16]. At least two case series have described pain relief with concurrent use of PNfS and SCS hybrid stimulation [17, 18]. Bernstein et al. [18] chronicled a series of 20 patients with combined SCS/PNfS with the majority of patients reporting a preference of the combined stimulation over either modality alone.

Currently, there are three large prospective studies investigating PNfS either alone or in combination with SCS. The two US studies are currently suspended, but in Europe there is a 200 patient study which is at present well over half enrolled [19]. McRoberts et al. [20] have published a prospective, randomized, controlled study of 44 patients with a year's follow-up. Excellent or good pain relief was reported by 68.2 % of patients at the 4-week visit, 69.5 % of patients at the 12-week visit, 60.8 % of patients at the 24-week visit, and again 69.5 % of patients at the 52-week visit. Also at the 52-week follow-up visit, 90.9 % ($N=20$) of patients indicated that they would undergo the procedure again, and 90.9 % ($N = 20$) of patients reported that they would recommend the procedure to a friend or family member. Visual analog score (VAS) was reduced from about 8/10 to less than 4/10 at the year mark. Kloimstein et al. [21] reported a multicenter, 118-patient prospective study of PNfS. They found that a mean VAS score at baseline of 7.9 reduced immediately to 4.58 after lead implantation and maintained at 4.7 at the end of the follow-up period of 6 months, yielding an average pain reduction of 44 %. Furthermore, at 6-month analysis, a mean opioid reduction from baseline of 69.4 % was achieved. A 2010 World Institute of Pain study followed 111 patients implanted with subcutaneous peripheral nerve stimulation [22] for a variety of conditions, the gross majority involving the axial cervical, thoracic, and lumbar areas. Pain intensity scores before and after subcutaneous target stimulation (STS) for all 111 patients yielded a median of 8/10 before STS and 4/10 after STS. A quarter of patients demonstrated a 75 % reduction in pain. In a 100 consecutive case series of PNfS published by Paul Verrills et al. [23], the majority of which focused on thoracic, lumbosacral, abdominal, pelvic, and groin pain, the average pain reduction was 7.4 to 3.2 on the VAS, at an 8.1-month follow-up. Well over half of patients rated either "good" or "excellent" pain relief, and less than 10 % were "unsatisfied" with their pain relief.

Implementation and Patient Selection

A familiarity with SCS is a first necessity. Multiple training courses exist for the surgeon to learn percutaneous implant techniques and the novice implanter is encouraged to attend several prior to attempting SCS, even if seasoned in the operating theater. It is essential to understand that success in pain relief with SCS, and even more so with PNS and HS, is predicated on an understanding of the usefulness of the neural target in mitigation of pain. Surgical technique predicts safety more than pain relief. The optimum patient describes truncal or cervical neuropathic pain that has been longstanding and unchanging. Yet unpublished retrospective data known to the author suggests, as does common sense, that pain syndromes that are often changing predict failure. The reprogramming plasticity of the implanted system is limited with SCS, and even more so with PNS, as smaller watersheds of paresthesia will simply be less likely to cover changing pain areas. The optimum patient describes long-term, unchanging pain.

Planning is essential, and involving the patient in the process crucial. Force the patient to draw on their bodies representations of their painful areas. Query and understand areas of maximal pain and most meaningful pain. Palpate and prod and generate a concept of depth and type of pain. Cognitively, the patient who does well with SCS is the same patient who does well with HS and PNfS; they understand the limitations of the therapy and have reasonable expectations and goals, and have been cleared by psychological assessment.

Summary

Axial pain syndromes greatly challenge the patient, surgeon, and interventionist for a variety of reasons. The sources of axial pain are often elusive, and even when identified often do not remit to surgical approaches. More rare than common is a painful, structural deformity which requires surgical fixation, and if performed is commonly plagued by painful syndromes in adjacent segments. The surgeries themselves produce traumatic results from which many patients never recover. In understanding the often profound challenges noted above, the concept of "hiding the pain from the brain" seems a more reasonable alternative. Traditional spinal cord stimulation has shown good effect in treating extremity pain, but is challenged in treating axial pain. While newer approaches, novel frequencies, and neural targets may improve outcomes in the low back, they too may be quite similarly challenged, as the aim of relief ascends the spine. Hybrid and PNfS may quite possibly remain the most favored and effective approach to treating axial pain in the neck and thoracic areas.

References

1. Krutsch JP, McCeney MH, Barolat G, et al. A case report of subcutaneous peripheral nerve stimulation for the treatment of axial back pain associated with postlaminectomy syndrome. Neuromodulation. 2008;12:112–5.
2. Gorosceniuk T, Koothari S. Targeted external area stimulation. Reg Anesth Pain Med. 2004;29 Suppl 2:98.
3. Lipov EG. Hybrid neurostimulator: simultaneous use of spinal cord and peripheral nerve field stimulation to treat low back and leg pain. Prog Neurol Surg. 2011;24:147–55.
4. North RB. Spinal cord and peripheral nerve stimulation: technical aspects. In: Simpson BA, editor. Pain research and clinical management. Electrical stimulation and the relief of pain. Philadelphia, PA: Elsevier; 2003. 15 (Chapter 12):183–96.
5. North RB, Ewend MG, Lawton MT, Piantadosi S. Spinal cord stimulation for chronic, intractable pain: superiority of "multi-channel" devices. Pain. 1991;44:119–30.
6. Sharan A, Cameron T, Barolat G. Evolving patterns of spinal cord stimulation in patients implanted for intractable low back and leg pain. Neuromodulation. 2002;5:167–79.
7. Feirabend HKP, Choufoer H, Ploeger S, Holsheimer J, van Gool JD. Morphometry of human superficial dorsal and dorsolateral column fibres: significance to spinal cord stimulation. Brain. 2002;125(5):1137–49.
8. Holsheimer J, Struijk JJ. How do geometric factors influence epidural spinal cord stimulation? A quantitative analysis by computer modeling. Stereotact Funct Neurosurg. 1991;56(4):234–49.
9. Haggqviat G, Lindberg J. On the size of the nucleus and cell in the spinal ganglia. Z Mikrosk Anat Forsch. 1961;67:529–51.
10. Alo KM, Holsheimer J. New trends in neuromodulation for the management of neuropathic pain. Neurosurgery. 2002;50:690–703.
11. Falco FJE, Berger J, Vrable A, Onyewu O, Zhu J. Cross talk: a new method for peripheral nerve stimulation. An observational report with cadaveric verification. Pain Physician. 2009;12:965–83.
12. Melzack R, Wall PD. Pain mechanisms: a new theory. Science. 1965;150:971–2.
13. Wall PD, Sweet WH. Temporary abolition of pain in man. Science. 1967;155:108–9.
14. Paicius RM, Bernstein CA, Lempert-Cohen C. Peripheral nerve field stimulation for the treatment of chronic low back pain: preliminary results of long-term follow-up—a case series. Neuromodulation. 2007;10:279–90.

15. Verrills P, Mitchell B, Vivian D, Sinclair C. Peripheral nerve stimulation: a treatment for chronic low back pain and failed back surgery syndrome? Neuromodulation. 2009;12:68–75.
16. Lipov EF, Joshi JR, Sanders S, Slavin KV. Use of peripheral subcutaneous field stimulation for the treatment of axial neck pain: a case report. Neuromodulation. 2009;12:292–5.
17. Lipov EG, Joshi JR, Slavin KV. Hybrid neuromodulation technique: use of combined spinal cord stimulation and peripheral nerve stimulation in treatment of chronic pain in back and legs. Acta Neurochir (Wien). 2008;150:971.
18. Bernstein CA, Paicius RM, Barkow SH, Lempert-Cohen C. Spinal cord stimulation in conjunction with peripheral nerve field stimulation for the treatment of low back and leg pain: a case series. Neuromodulation. 2008;11:116–23.
19. Eldabe Sam. Email communication to W. Porter McRoberts. 28 May 2015.
20. McRoberts WP, Wolkowitz R, Meyer DJ, Lipov E, Joshi J, Davis B, Cairns KD, Barolat G. Peripheral nerve field stimulation for the management of localized chronic intractable back pain: results from a randomized controlled study. Neuromodulation. 2013;16:565–75.
21. Kloimstein H, Likar R, Kern M, Neuhold J, Cada M, Loinig N, Ilias W, Freundl B, Binder H, Wolf A, Dorn C, Mozes-Balla EM, Stein R, Lappe I, Sator-Katzenschlager S. Peripheral nerve field stimulation (PNFS) in chronic low back pain: a prospective multicenter study. Neuromodulation. 2014;17:180–7.
22. Sator-Katzenschlager SS, Fiala K, Kress HG, Kofler A, Neuhold J, Kloimstein H, Ilias W, Mozes-Balla E, Pinter M, Loining N, Fuchs W, Heinze G, Likar R. Subcutaneous target stimulation (STS) in chronic noncancer pain: a nationwide retrospective study. Pain Pract. 2010;10(4):279–86.
23. Verrills P, et al. Peripheral nerve field stimulation for chronic pain: 100 cases and review of the literature. Pain Med. 2011;12:1395–405.

Chapter 19
Intrathecal Drug Delivery: Surgical Technique

William S. Rosenberg

Key Points

- Good preoperative understanding of the patient's diagnosis and disease process, pain distribution, anticipated future treatments, and preferences is required.
- Meticulous attention to surgical detail and tissue handling is necessary for good outcomes and a low infection rate.
- A tunneled, externalized intrathecal catheter can be a simple, successful, and cost-effective way to control pain in palliative care or end-of-life circumstances.
- Epidural hematoma and spinal cord injury must be ruled out in the case of new, immediate postoperative neurological deficit that is not rapidly responsive to changes in intrathecal dosing.
- A new neurological deficit in a chronically implanted intrathecal drug delivery system must raise the concern for inflammatory mass.
- An infected intrathecal drug delivery system must be removed, except under unusual circumstances involving short-term life expectancy.

Introduction

Intrathecal drug delivery can be a life-changing intervention for the patient with chronic or cancer-related pain. The spine surgeon is well suited to take part in any or all the steps ranging from implementation, maintenance, and troubleshooting such a system, in addition to participating in patient selection

W.S. Rosenberg, M.D., F.A.A.N.S. (✉)
Center for the Relief of Pain, Midwest Neuroscience Institute,
2330 East Meyer Blvd., Suite 411, Kansas City, MO 64132, USA
e-mail: wsr@post.harvard.edu

© Springer International Publishing Switzerland 2016　　　　　　211
S.M. Falowski, J.E. Pope (eds.), *Integrating Pain Treatment into Your Spine Practice*, DOI 10.1007/978-3-319-27796-7_19

and ongoing treatment, if interested. Complete understanding of the device, its implantation, and use in treating pain is necessary for good patient outcomes.

Patient Selection

From the surgeon's perspective, patient selection often begins with the referring physician and the broader issues of determining the proper patient for implantation will be covered elsewhere in this publication. However, regardless of whether the recommendation for intrathecal drug delivery (IDD) is originating elsewhere, it is incumbent on the implanting surgeon to develop a complete understanding of the patient's diagnosis, natural history, overall treatment plan, and any concurrent medical issues. Often patients will have multiple painful areas and it is important to achieve a clear consensus with the patient (and referring physician, if applicable) as to the exact distribution of the pain for which IDD is being used. Active infection is almost always a contraindication to initiating IDD and this diagnosis must be sought and actively treated prior to implantation. Similarly, coagulopathy—whether pathological or iatrogenic—must be addressed. A careful physical examination is required, in particular to document any existing findings that might be confusing after implantation.

It is important to verify the patient's understanding of IDD and his/her comfort with the concept and procedure. While the referring physician may have primary responsibility for recommending and managing IDD, the surgeon, by virtue of implanting the device, becomes part of that patient's health care team. Failure to achieve consensus on the realistic issues of life with an IDD system and reasonable goals for pain control can result in postoperative symptoms (e.g., pump-related discomfort) that can and will involve the implanting surgeon. These can often be mitigated through preoperative education and agreement. Moreover, it is important to have an understanding of, and to fully engage, the patient's social support systems and infrastructure in this education, thereby increasing the likelihood of successful treatment.

The issue of intrathecal drug trialing in patient selection is complex and will be covered more extensively in other chapters. In short, if trialing is desired, it can be achieved using several different paradigms: single injection, temporary epidural or intrathecal catheter, or permanent intrathecal catheter [1]. If the latter is desired—in which the intrathecal catheter that is placed is the one that will be used for long-term, pump-delivered treatment—this procedure is discussed below under tunneled, externalized catheter for palliation. In any event, the delivery of an intraspinal opioid dose mandates at least 24 h of observation for respiratory compromise to avoid serious complication.

Technique

Preoperative Planning

Prior to arriving in the operating room, it is important to have determined the desired spinal level of the intrathecal catheter and the planned location of the pump pocket.

The appropriate level for catheter placement will be determined by the distribution of the pain that requires coverage. Since CSF flow and drug distribution are practically limited to several spinal levels above and below the catheter tip, optimal surgical planning requires careful consideration of this dermatomal distribution [2]. It is important to be realistic in the number of dermatomes that can be covered and to consider other treatment modalities if the required coverage is too extensive. For head and neck analgesia, placement of the catheter tip in the high cervical canal or even foramen magnum can be successful. For lower back pain, placement of the catheter tip in the mid to lower thoracic region is usually desired.

The factors influencing pump pocket placement are (1) body habitus, (2) natural history of the disease process, (3) anticipated future treatments, and (4) patient preference. While it is very important to anchor the pump to fascia in order to prevent flipping and refill problems, competing with this is the requirement for placement close enough to the skin surface to allow for pump interrogation and needle access. The body habitus of some obese patients with thick subcutaneous fat may preclude fulfilling both of these requirements at the usual abdominal location. In addition, the usual abdominal pump pocket location may need to be modified because of stomas, drains, and other issues impacting the abdominal wall.

Particularly in the case of cancer-related pain, the natural progression of the disease, as well as anticipated future treatments, must be considered. Since the liver is often involved, or becomes involved, with metastatic cancer, a right upper quadrant pump placement is best avoided, if possible. Placement in this location will preclude adequate clinical evaluation and sometimes treatment. With radiotherapy, for example, the pump should not be located directly in the radiation beam. If radiation treatment is currently being employed or anticipated for the future, coordination with the radiation oncologist is mandatory in optimal surgical planning [3].

The location of the pump pocket should be planned by the surgeon, with active patient participation, in the preoperative holding area. Relevant positions, such as sitting, should be explored and contact with an osseous surface (e.g., rib or anterior iliac crest) should be avoided, as this will result in chronic postoperative pain. For complex situations, alternative locations to the abdomen can include the lateral chest wall on the thoracic ribs in the posterior axillary line, the buttock region, or the medial thigh. The lateral chest wall can be a good location for obese patients whose abdominal subcutaneous fat prevents acceptably securing the pump.

Patient Positioning

The usual position for placement of the pump in the abdomen or chest wall is lateral decubitus. It is important to verify that there is no obstruction to fluoroscopic visualization along the entire anticipated course of the intrathecal catheter. This is particularly important for cervical placement. It can be very helpful to make sure that both the thoracic and lumbar spine are perpendicular to the floor when positioning on the operative table, which usually requires building up the padding between the arms until the upper arm is parallel to the floor and securing the thorax and hips with wide tape. For upper thoracic and cervical catheter placement, care must be taken to position the arms in such a way that they do not interfere with fluoroscopy.

Catheter Placement

The intrathecal catheter is usually placed via paramedian approach through a Tuohy needle, as this approach has been demonstrated to result in a lower incidence of catheter breakage than an interspinous midline trajectory. It is important to plan the needle track to achieve the shallowest angle of incidence as is practical. This will allow more translation of driving force along the longitudinal axis of the catheter and, thus, result in easier placement, as well as reduced complications such as occlusion and breakage.

Once the entry site for the needle is selected, a small incision is made and taken down to the lumbar fascia. Clear visualization of the fascia is important to assure adequate anchoring (see below). The Tuohy needle is then placed into the thecal sac. Once there is the free flow of CSF, the pump is opened and prepared by the scrub tech on the back table, thereby preventing unnecessary expense if placement of the catheter proves impossible. Fluoroscopy can be helpful in placing the catheter, particularly in obese patients. Many implanters place a purse-string suture in the fascia around the catheter entry site. Placement of this purse-string suture, as well as incising the fascia to accommodate a transfascial anchor, is most safely performed with the Tuohy needle in place (Fig. 19.1).

Once the fascial entry site is prepared, the intrathecal catheter is placed under fluoroscopic guidance (Fig. 19.2). The ideal location of the catheter tip is dorsal to the spinal cord. Frequently, placement is quite smooth and the proper spinal level is easily attained. However, it is useful to know strategies for those cases in which this is not the case. The CSF space changes with the cardiac cycle. Sometimes, attempting to advance the catheter in time with the audible pulse oximeter can allow the catheter to advance during the phase of maximal thecal sac diameter. Another technique involves gross manipulation of the patient's shoulder in a dorsoventral plane while advancing the catheter, changing the orientation of the catheter within the thecal sac and sometimes allowing it to pass through an area of obstruction. Lastly, spinning the hub of the catheter—with or without placing a small bend in the tip of

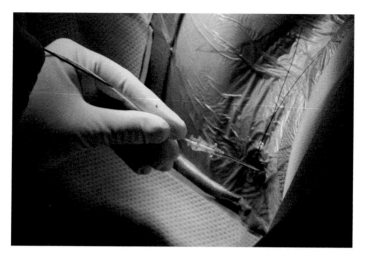

Fig. 19.1 Placement of intrathecal catheter through Tuohy needle after accessing CSF. Note: Black suture is purse-string placed around needle as it passes through fascia which, at this point, remains untied

Fig. 19.2 Radio-opaque intrathecal catheter after cervical placement

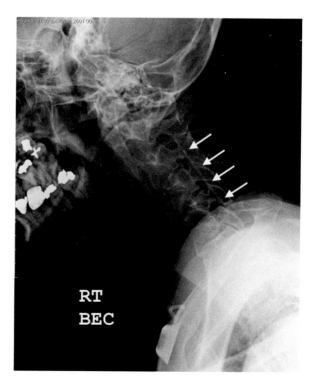

the stylet—can sometimes allow the catheter to find a path through the obstruction. Once the catheter tip is at the appropriate level, the stylet and needle are withdrawn and intrathecal placement, if needed, is verified using contrast (e.g., iohexol) and subtraction fluoroscopy.

Pump Pocket and Tunneling

In creating the pump pocket, it is important to maintain the manufacturer-recommended depth from the skin surface to facilitate communication and refills. If at all possible, it is optimal to expose the pocket along the fascia to allow for adequate anchoring, thereby preventing "flipping" of the pump. Meticulous hemostasis is required to reduce the incidence of pocket hematoma. Once this has been achieved, four non-absorbable sutures are placed in the quadrants of the pocket, secured to the fascia. The catheter is tunneled subcutaneously into the pump pocket with care to maintain a subcutaneous level. Too shallow placement can result in pain and erosion; too deep placement when tunneling between the back and the abdomen can result in soft tissue injury and/or entry into the peritoneal cavity (see below).

Once the catheter is in the pump pocket, the pump is attached to its proximal end and placed into the pocket (Fig. 19.3). Excess catheter is coiled underneath the pump to reduce the possibility of damaging it during pump needle access. Vancomycin powder can be placed prior to pump placement (see below). Once the pump and catheter are in their final position, the catheter is accessed using the appropriate needle and the proper port and enough CSF are withdrawn to confirm catheter patency and empty it of any residual dye. A multilayered, tension-free

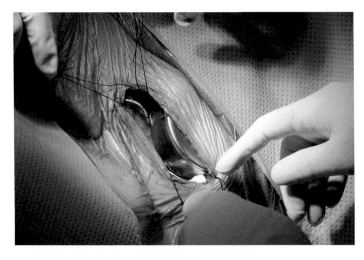

Fig. 19.3 Pump within pump pocket. Anchoring sutures are being tied

closure is performed on both the pocket and the catheter incision, with particular attention to a watertight closure of the lumbar incision.

Infection Prevention

Infection of an IDD system is a potentially preventable complication that can have devastating consequences. Not only is there significant clinical risk, possibly including meningitis, but there are also psychological consequences of having to remove a successful implant and the economic costs of ultimately replacing the system. Therefore, infection prevention is exceedingly important.

The mainstay of infection prevention, as is true for most surgical procedures, is meticulous attention to tissue handling, hemostasis, and closure. Preoperative antibiotics should be dosed and timed appropriately. Excessive cautery, resulting in retained dead tissue, should be avoided. An iodine-impregnated surgical adhesive drape should be used, as well as silver-impregnated surgical bandages.

There are several low-cost techniques that will almost certainly result in a lower infection rate, although no high-quality clinical data on these strategies have been collected. Frequent and copious irrigation with antibiotic solution is recommended, along with stapling antibiotic-soaked sponges to the skin edges of each incision prior to placing any material that will remain in the body after closure. Vancomycin powder is inexpensive and can be used in both the pump pocket and catheter incision.

Revision Strategies

Revision of an IDD system can range from a simple pump replacement to a diagnostic exploration. The general principles are the same as with primary implantation. Low-energy electrocautery can be quite helpful and expeditious in dissecting out catheter embedded in scar without damaging it. At times, it may be necessary to place a new intrathecal catheter, in which case the prior catheter can be tied off and left in place, avoiding the significant risk of persistent CSF leak if it is removed. If removal is necessary and the track to the dura is persistent, fibrin glue injection down that track prior to closing it can be helpful in preventing a CSF leak.

Documentation

Adequate documentation of the implant procedure is necessary, both to provide information to the implanter in the future and to provide a new health care provider with enough information to care for the patient. Minimally, the operative note should include the precise system being implanted, the final spinal level of the catheter tip, and whether it is dorsal or ventral to the spinal cord. This latter information can be important in interpreting new neurological symptoms. This same information, along with the name of the implanter and date of implantation, can often also be placed into memory on the pump, providing an emergency backup if the operative note is unavailable.

Special Circumstances

Tunneled Externalized Catheter for Palliation

For end-of-life palliation, as well as for permanent catheter trials (see above), it may be desirable to place an externalized, tunneled intrathecal catheter and connect it to an external pump [4, 5]. This can be very cost effective when the patient's life expectancy is short and, if done properly, can be internalized to an implanted pump if the clinical situation significantly changes (or the trial is successful).

The catheter implantation procedure for an externalized catheter is described above. A small incision is made in another area, often a smaller incision along the course of that which would be used for pump placement, if applicable. The catheter is tunneled subcutaneously into the second field; an extension is attached, brought out through a separate stab incision, and attached to a pump. Attachment of the catheter to the external pump tubing can be challenging and require ingenuity, as there is no standard system for achieving this.

If pump implantation is desired, the anticipated pump incision is prepped and the exit site of the catheter is draped out of the field. The pump incision is made, the catheter exposed, and the extension disconnected and removed by the circulating nurse from outside the sterile field. Implantation of the pump can then proceed as usual.

Open Catheter Placement via Laminotomy

On rare occasion, placement of an intrathecal catheter using a needle-based technique is impossible. If warranted, a catheter can be placed under direct visualization via laminotomy using standard neurosurgical principles. In such cases, a purse-string suture in the dura around the catheter can often help to prevent persistent CSF leak.

C1/2 Puncture for Catheter Placement

Even less common are cases requiring placement of the catheter through a C1/2 puncture (Fig. 19.4). The principles as outlined above are similar, although steering the catheter caudally to the desired level can be challenging because of the necessary perpendicular angle of the needle.

Fig. 19.4 C1/2 placement of intrathecal catheter. The catheter can be seen exiting the needle (*black arrows*) and being placed caudally to the T1/2 level (*inset, blue arrows*)

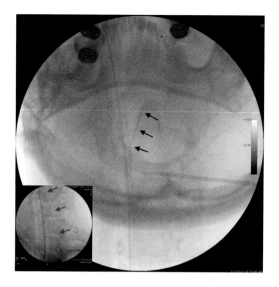

Troubleshooting and Complication Management

Neurological Deterioration

A new neurological deficit immediately following routine placement of an IDD system is rare and underscores the importance of a careful, well-documented preoperative neurological assessment. Depending on the nature of the new finding, an MRI can usually rapidly address the unlikely possibility of an epidural hematoma or spinal cord injury. Once these possibilities are eliminated, one can focus on the more likely scenario of drug effect from the newly administered intrathecal medication.

A new neurological deficit in a chronically implanted IDD system should raise the prospect of a catheter-associated inflammatory mass (see below).

CSF Leak

On occasion, patients will develop the signs and symptoms of a CSF leak following IDD system implantation. An actual leak through the suture line needs to be immediately addressed to prevent egress of CSF and the consequent potential for dehiscence and/or infection. Postural headache with or without nausea and vomiting, in the absence of visible CSF leakage, can often be treated using noninvasive modalities. Rest with limitation of upright posture, analgesics, caffeine, and hydration can often ameliorate the CSF leak, although the time required to maintain such therapy is frequently longer than is the case without an intrathecal catheter. If the CSF leak persists, a percutaneous blood patch or surgical exploration should be considered.

Infection

In almost all cases, documented infection of an IDD system requires complete removal of the implant, as the risk of meningitis can be high. Reimplantation can certainly be considered once appropriate antibiotic therapy has been administered, possibly at another pump pocket site. If the causal organism is in doubt, cultures can be obtained at the time of explantation, and CSF can be collected from the catheter for examination prior to withdrawal if there is concern for meningitis.

One exception to immediate implant removal is in the case of highly effective intrathecal analgesia and very short life expectancy. In such cases, the benefit of maintaining pain control and quality of life in the short term may outweigh the risk of progressive infection. Paradoxically, this is most true when the pump pocket is draining or even partially open. Under those circumstances, there is no risk of abscess formation with pressure driving infection along the catheter and toward the intrathecal space. As long as the open pocket can be adequately managed with dressings, this situation can be maintained at the end of life, even for months, if necessary. There have been reports of salvaging infected pumps using various antibiotic-impregnated delivery mechanisms within the pocket [6].

Pump Malfunction

The implanting surgeon may be asked to participate in the evaluation of a pump malfunction. This can present as sudden loss of clinical efficacy, intermittent symptom of over- or underdosage, or with a more overt sign, such as fluid accumulation in the pump pocket. A methodical approach to this diagnosis is valuable, as failure modes exist throughout the system.

When confronted with a patient in whom clinical efficacy of the intrathecal drug delivery is being questioned, and if there is a local anesthetic in the pump (e.g., bupivacaine), a very useful office test for overall drug delivery and efficacy can be a one-time, supervised bolus. A bolus of 1–2 mg bupivacaine over a short time period (1–2 min) will produce a limited regional anesthetic effect (sensory level, motor weakness) consistent with the level of the catheter tip. Because of these effects, this test should NOT be performed if the catheter tip is in the cervical spine, as there is a risk of respiratory compromise. The patient is requested to completely empty his/her urinary bladder prior to the bolus, as short-term urinary retention can result. In addition, a warning is given with regard to probable lower extremity weakness to avoid patient distress and the bolus is given after the patient is placed in a comfortable recumbent position. If the clinical findings after the bolus are consistent with the record of catheter placement, the pump has been confirmed to be delivering medication to the appropriate level and consideration should be made for adjusting the dose and/or medication.

A useful start in assessing a possible pump malfunction is to interrogate the device and examine the logs stored on it. One might find that the pump is, in fact, near the end of its anticipated life and should be replaced. Alternatively, a pattern of motor stalls or other complications may help in identifying the problem. If a motor stall is correlated with exposure to high-strength magnetic fields (e.g., MRI), this might reflect the normal functioning of the pump. Unexplained motor stalls, especially if they occur with some frequency, are not normal and need to be investigated.

If there are symptoms of underdosage just prior to refill and/or overdosage just after refill, careful determination of the actual reservoir volume should be performed and compared to the anticipated volume. This comparison should be a routine component of the refill procedure and recorded. Any significant discrepancy needs to be investigated. This can be done by performing a comparison within a few days of refill. If there is concern for risk to the patient, the medication can be replaced with saline while the pump is being investigated. If this approach is taken, depending on the clinical scenario, the patient should be covered with systemic medication to prevent a withdrawal syndrome.

If there is further concern for pump malfunction, serial fluoroscopic examination of the pump can be performed with attention to the positioning of the rotor ("rotor study"). This is often done in conjunction with the placement of intrathecal dye within the pump (see below).

Catheter Complications

Another etiology for loss of clinical efficacy can be related to catheter malfunction. The catheter can become disrupted or disconnected, causing diversion of medication. It can change spinal levels, producing deviations in clinical effects, or become blocked or kinked, causing complete failure of medication egress.

If the patency or connectivity of the catheter is in question, the easiest, fastest, and most cost-effective way to assess the catheter is using an in-office bolus (see above), if possible. If this approach is not possible, a catheter study can be performed under fluoroscopic guidance. The catheter is accessed percutaneously and enough CSF is withdrawn to clear it of medication. This step is critical as failure to clear the catheter could result in an injurious and potentially fatal intrathecal bolus of medication during infusion of contrast. (The inability to withdraw CSF, however, is not itself an indication of catheter malfunction.) Once the catheter is filled with CSF, intrathecal contrast can be instilled and followed radiographically. One study used high-resolution 3D computed tomography to diagnose a catheter leak that was not apparent on fluoroscopy [7].

Another cause of loss of efficacy or need for frequent dosage increases is the formation of an inflammatory mass at the catheter tip [8]. Formerly known as a "granuloma," its presentation can range from dosing and efficacy issues as described to frank neurological deficit associated with a compressive intradural extramedullary mass lesion (Fig. 19.5), underscoring the importance of a careful neurological examination during pump refills. If there is no neurological deficit, an inflammatory mass will often involute in response to changing to saline intrathecal delivery and/or repositioning the catheter tip. If the presence of neurological deficits precludes waiting for regression, surgical resection and decompression can be considered (Fig. 19.6). The risks and benefits of this approach need to be carefully weighed,

Fig. 19.5 Thoracic
CT-myelogram showing
inflammatory mass
surrounding two intrathecal
catheters. Spinal cord is
displaced to the right and
posteriorly

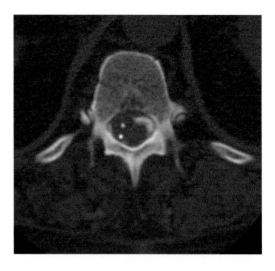

Fig. 19.6 Intraoperative
ultrasound through dura
after laminectomy. *Asterisk*
marks the inflammatory
mass with the more
hypoechoic spinal cord
rotated upward and to the
left

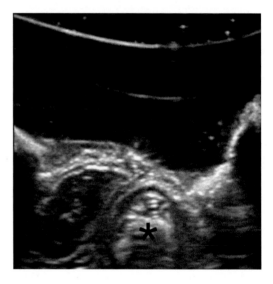

however, as there can be dense adhesions to the surrounding structures, including
the spinal cord and nerve roots, increasing the risk of neurological injury. Standard
neurosurgical techniques are used (Fig. 19.7) and the catheter can be repositioned,
removed, or replaced as appropriate.

A rare complication of intrathecal catheter placement is peritoneal transgres-
sion during subcutaneous passage between a lumbar operative site and an
abdominal pump pocket (Fig. 19.8). This warrants particular consideration in
debilitated patients, such as those with extensive cancer, and can occur in all

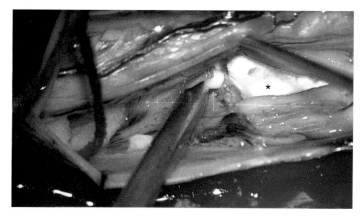

Fig. 19.7 Intraoperative microphotograph of conus (*across top*) displaced by partially resected inflammatory mass. Note: *Blue arrow* indicates the visible portion of catheter within the mass that ends in a crystallized accumulation of intrathecal medication (*asterisk*)

Fig. 19.8 Abdominal CT scan with intraperitoneal catheter (*blue arrow*)

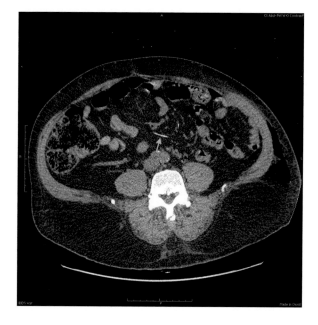

types of patient body habitus. A small through-and-through entry into the peritoneal cavity can result in the eventual location of almost the entire catheter within the peritoneum as a result of the negative pressure. The catheter can be revised with gentle, steady pressure, withdrawing it from within the peritoneum and abdominal exploration is rarely required, as long as no visceral injury has occurred.

Pump Pocket Complications

A fluid collection can form around the pump in the subcutaneous pocket. Wearing an abdominal binder for several weeks following implantation can sometimes mitigate this seroma. It requires treatment only if (a) it becomes painful or physically unmanageable or (b) it interferes with normally interrogating and refilling the pump. In this rare event, sterile percutaneous aspiration is often curative. If the problem does not resolve with one or two aspirations, catheter fracture or another mechanism causing CSF accumulation should be considered. In the case of recurrent seroma refractory to multiple drainage attempts and other treatments, doxycycline sclerotherapy can be used [9].

A pump that has not been adequately secured or has come loose from anchoring can be quite mobile within the pocket, at times completely turning over such that there is no longer percutaneous access—the "flipped" pump. This is a major problem as it both impedes the ability to interrogate and communicate with the pump and completely prevents refilling it. The latter can be an urgent clinical problem in cases of very low reserve medication. Sometimes it is possible to manipulate the pump to flip back over into the normal position, using gentle but steady manual pressure. This can save the patient from an emergency surgery in the case of urgent need to refill the pump. The only other option is to explore the pump pocket and surgically reposition and restabilize the pump.

Summary

The spine surgeon can, and should, be an integral member of the team implementing and managing intrathecal drug delivery. The surgical skill set is well used in the implantation and maintenance of these complex devices. Thoughtful and well-considered diagnosis, artful technique, and sound understanding of fundamental clinical principles are critical in the service of achieving the best and longest lasting pain relief possible for the patient.

References

1. Deer TR, Prager J, Levy R, et al. Polyanalgesic consensus conference-2012: recommendations on trialing for intrathecal (intraspinal) drug delivery: report of an interdisciplinary expert panel. Neuromodulation. 2012;15:420–35.
2. Deer TR, Prager J, Levy R, et al. Polyanalgesic consensus conference 2012: recommendations for the management of pain by intrathecal (intraspinal) drug delivery: report of an interdisciplinary expert panel. Neuromodulation. 2012;15:436–66.
3. Gebhardt R, Ludwig M, Kirsner S, Kosturakis AK. Implanted intrathecal drug delivery systems and radiation treatment. Pain Med. 2013;14:398–402.

4. Aprili D, Bandschapp O, Rochlitz C, Urwyler A, Ruppen W. Serious complications associated with external intrathecal catheters used in cancer pain patients: a systematic review and meta-analysis. Anesthesiology. 2009;111:1346–55.
5. Wilkes D, Cook M, Solanki D. Intrathecal catheter-syringe adaptor for short-term intrathecal analgesia with an externalized pump: a case report. Pain Physician. 2010;13:151–6.
6. Peerdeman SM, de Groot V, Feller RE. In situ treatment of an infected intrathecal baclofen pump implant with gentamicin-impregnated collagen fleece. J Neurosurg. 2010;112:1308–10.
7. Ellis JA, Leung R, Winfree CJ. Spinal infusion pump-catheter leak detected by high-resolution 3D computed tomography. J Neurosurg Spine. 2011;15:555–7.
8. Deer TR, Prager J, Levy R, et al. Polyanalgesic consensus conference-2012: consensus on diagnosis, detection, and treatment of catheter-tip granulomas (inflammatory masses). Neuromodulation. 2012;15:483–96.
9. Caliendo MV, Lee DE, Queiroz R, Waldman DL. Sclerotherapy with use of doxycycline after percutaneous drainage of postoperative lymphoceles. J Vasc Interv Radiol. 2001;12:73–7.

Chapter 20
Vertebroplasty and Kyphoplasty

Ronil V. Chandra, Tony Goldschlager, Thabele M. Leslie-Mazwi,
and Joshua A. Hirsch

Key Points

- Vertebroplasty and kyphoplasty are image-guided, minimally invasive procedures that involve injection of cement into a fractured vertebral body.
- The primary goal of vertebroplasty and kyphoplasty is reduction in back pain and disability.
- For selected patients with cancer and disabling back pain from a vertebral fracture, kyphoplasty is superior to conservative medical therapy in reducing back pain, disability, and improving quality of life for patients. Both vertebroplasty and kyphoplasty are reasonable treatments in selected patients with cancer and disabling back pain from a vertebral fracture that is refractory to conservative medical therapy.

R.V. Chandra, M.B.B.S., M.Med., F.R.A.N.Z.C.R. (✉)
Monash Imaging, Monash Health, 246 Clayton Road, Clayton,
Melbourne, VIC 3168, Australia

Department of Surgery, Monash University, Melbourne, VIC, Australia
e-mail: Ronil.Chandra@monashhealth.org

T. Goldschlager, M.B.B.S., Ph.D., F.R.A.C.S.
Department of Surgery, Monash University, Melbourne, VIC, Australia

Department of Neurosurgery, Monash Health,
246 Clayton Road, Clayton, Melbourne, VIC 3168, Australia
e-mail: Tony.Goldschlager@monashhealth.org

T.M. Leslie-Mazwi, M.D. • J.A. Hirsch, M.D., F.A.C.R., F.S.I.R.
NeuroInterventional Program, Massachusetts General Hospital,
Harvard Medical School, 55 Fruit St., GRB 2-241, Boston, MA 02114, USA
e-mail: TLeslie-Mazwi@mgh.harvard.edu; JAHirsch@mgh.harvard.edu

© Springer International Publishing Switzerland 2016
S.M. Falowski, J.E. Pope (eds.), *Integrating Pain Treatment into Your Spine Practice*, DOI 10.1007/978-3-319-27796-7_20

227

- For selected patients with osteoporosis and disabling back pain from a vertebral fracture, there is conflicting data from randomized controlled trials. Overall, both vertebroplasty and kyphoplasty are reasonable treatments in selected patients with osteoporosis and disabling back pain from a vertebral fracture that is refractory to conservative medical therapy.
- Complications from performing vertebroplasty and kyphoplasty are uncommon and are generally caused by extra-osseous leakage of the injected cement that may go unrecognized by the operator in real time. This may cause local radiculopathy, lower extremity paralysis, and/or distal embolism. These risks can be minimized by strict adherence to meticulous technique and a conservative treatment strategy.

Introduction

Vertebroplasty and kyphoplasty are image-guided minimally invasive procedures that involve injection of an implant, most typically cement, into a fractured vertebral body. While vertebroplasty involves injection of cement directly after introduction of a percutaneous needle into the vertebral body, kyphoplasty involves an additional step in which a cavity is created, most typically by inflating a balloon tamp within the vertebral body into which the cement is subsequently injected. These procedures are performed to relieve back pain and disability from symptomatic osteoporotic or neoplasm-related vertebral compression fractures that are refractory to conservative medical therapy.

Osteoporotic Vertebral Fractures

The majority of osteoporotic vertebral fractures are asymptomatic, or result in tolerable symptoms. Only a third of new fractures result in medical attention [1]. In most patients, the resulting acute back pain resolves over 6–8 weeks as the fracture heals [2]. These patients are typically managed with oral analgesics and/or bed rest, as well as orthotic devices and physical therapy. Calcium and vitamin D supplementation and anti-resorptive agents also aid in prevention of future vertebral fractures. Conservative medical management is appropriate for patients with mild pain and disability; however for patients with severe pain and marked disability, conservative treatment is not benign. In this cohort, high-dose narcotics may lead to undesirable side effects such as excessive sedation, and bed rest can lead to loss of bone mass and deconditioning. These ill effects are particularly pronounced in elderly patients. Such patients may benefit from vertebroplasty or kyphoplasty to facilitate more rapid pain relief and improvement in functional status compared with ongoing conservative medical management.

Neoplasm-Related Vertebral Fractures

Patients with spinal neoplasms commonly experience back pain. Stretching or invasion of the periosteum can cause local pain, while foraminal or epidural tumors may cause neural dysfunction and/or neuropathic pain. Osteolytic tumor deposits weaken bony integrity, and secondary vertebral compression fracture can acutely exacerbate back pain. This is particularly evident in multiple myeloma where one in three patients will experience a painful vertebral fracture [3]. Conservative medical management remains the mainstay of treatment, with palliative radiotherapy as an effective adjunctive treatment. However new or worsening vertebral fractures occur in up to a third of patients after spinal radiotherapy [4–6], and the total dose is limited by the tolerance of adjacent tissues, in particular the spinal cord. For such patients with neoplasm-related vertebral fractures, vertebroplasty and kyphoplasty offer additional treatment options to facilitate rapid pain relief and improvement in functional status. In addition, these treatments may provide additional structural support preventing further vertebral collapse.

Evidence

Integrating the best available evidence from the medical literature with clinician expertise whilst accounting for patient values allows for best evidence-based clinical practice. Since the publication of the two highly publicized negative randomized controlled trials of vertebroplasty for osteoporotic fracture in the New England Journal of Medicine in 2009, subsequent larger prospective randomized controlled trials have provided further high-quality evidence to guide current clinical practice; outcomes of the major prospective randomized controlled trials for vertebroplasty and kyphoplasty are summarized below.

The INVEST (*Investigational Vertebroplasty Safety and Efficacy Trial*) published in the *New England Journal of Medicine* in 2009 was a prospective international multicenter randomized "sham-controlled" trial of vertebroplasty for osteoporotic fracture [7]. Patients were included if back pain intensity was scored 3 or more (scale 0–10) with less than 12-month duration with failure of pain relief with conservative medical therapy. If fracture age was uncertain, bone marrow edema on MRI or increased activity on bone scan was required. A total of 131 patients were randomized to vertebroplasty ($n=68$) or "sham" procedure groups ($n=63$). At baseline, mean back pain intensity was 7 and duration was 16 weeks in the vertebroplasty group and 18 weeks in the control group. Mean modified Roland–Morris Disability Questionnaire (RDQ) score was 17 in the vertebroplasty group and 18 in the control group indicating significant disability. At 1 month, there was no difference in the primary outcome measures of back pain intensity or RDQ score ($P=0.19$ and $P=0.49$, respectively). Some of the major limitations of the INVEST trial were inclusion of fractures up to 12 months old (pain for >6 months was present in one-third of patients), the lack of a physical examination component, lack of MRI or bone scan as part of the inclusion criteria, and the use of a controlled intervention rather than a true sham.

An Australian prospective multicenter blinded randomized sham-controlled trial of vertebroplasty for osteoporotic fracture was also published in the *New England Journal of Medicine* in 2009 [8]. Patients were included if there was back pain of less than 12-month duration and recent vertebral fracture as defined by vertebral collapse, a fracture line, and/or bone marrow edema. A total of 78 patients were randomized to vertebroplasty ($n=38$) or sham procedure ($n=40$) groups. At baseline, average back pain intensity was 7 and duration of 9 weeks in both groups. At 3 months, there was no difference in the primary outcome measure of overall back pain intensity. Some of the major limitations included inclusion of fractures up to 12 months old (pain>6 weeks was present for 70 % of patients), the lack of a minimum back pain score, the lack of a physical examination component, and small patient numbers.

The Fracture Reduction Evaluation (FREE) trial was a prospective international multicenter open-label randomized conservative management controlled trial of kyphoplasty for osteoporotic fractures also published in 2009 [9]. Patients were included if there was back pain of less than 3-month duration, with a score of 4 or more (scale 0–10) and vertebral bone marrow edema or pseudoarthrosis on MRI scans. A total of 300 patients were randomized into kyphoplasty ($n=149$) or conservative medical management groups ($n=151$). At baseline, mean duration of back pain was approximately 6 weeks. Mean time between randomization and kyphoplasty was 7 days. By 1 month, kyphoplasty resulted in significantly improved quality of life over conservative management, achieving the primary outcome measure ($P<0.0001$). In addition, back pain scores were significantly reduced at 1 week ($P<0.0001$) and 12 months ($P=0.0034$). Limitations of the FREE trial included the lack of blinding which can overestimate treatment benefit, and the inclusion of a small number of neoplasm-related fractures ($n=4$).

The VERTOS II trial published in 2010 was a prospective international multicenter open-label randomized conservative management controlled trial of vertebroplasty for osteoporotic fracture published [10]. Patients were included if there was severe back pain with visual analogue scale (VAS) score of 5 or more, for less than 6-week duration, focal tenderness on physical examination at the fractured level, and bone marrow edema on MRI scan. A total of 202 patients were randomized into vertebroplasty ($n=101$) or conservative medical management ($n=101$) groups. At baseline, mean VAS scores were 7.8 and 7.5 in the respective groups for a mean of 30 days. Vertebroplasty resulted in significantly greater pain relief at 1 month than conservative treatment, meeting the primary outcome measure. The mean reduction of VAS score from baseline was 2.6 greater in the vertebroplasty group ($P<0.0001$). This was a durable effect with a significant difference between groups in favor of vertebroplasty at 1 year. Notable secondary outcomes were earlier significant pain (reduction in VAS by 3 or more) relief in the vertebroplasty group (30 days vs. 116 days, $P<0.0001$) and a gain in 120 pain-free (VAS 0–3) in the 12 months after vertebroplasty. A major limitation in the VERTOS II trial was a lack of blinding which can overestimate treatment effect.

The Cancer Patient Fracture Evaluation (CAFE) trial published in 2011 was a prospective international multicenter open-label randomized conservative management controlled trial of kyphoplasty for fractures in cancer patients [11]. Patients were included if back pain score was 4 or more (scale 0–10) and RDQ disability score of 10 or more from a clinically diagnosed vertebral fracture in a patient with cancer; fractures were confirmed with plain radiography or MRI. A total of 134 patients were randomized into kyphoplasty ($n=70$) or conservative therapy groups ($n=64$). At baseline, estimated symptomatic fracture age was 3.5 months; 70 % of patients had edema on MRI. Mean baseline RDQ scores were 18 points in both groups indicating severe disability. Kyphoplasty resulted in significantly greater reduction in back pain-related disability than conservative management, meeting the primary outcome measure. The treatment effect for kyphoplasty was 8.4 points ($P<0.0001$). Notable secondary outcomes included significant reduction of back pain after 7 days in the kyphoplasty group, but no change in the conservative management group ($P<0.0001$), as well as significant improvements in Karnofsky performance status score after 1 month in the kyphoplasty group but no significant change in the conservative management group ($P<0.0001$). Limitations of the CAFE trials include the lack of histological confirmation of vertebral fracture etiology. Thus fractures may have been caused by metastasis, radionecrosis, osteoporosis, or a combination.

Subsequent meta-analyses of prospective randomized and non-randomized controlled trials comparing vertebroplasty and kyphoplasty to conservative or sham treatment for osteoporotic fractures were subsequently published in 2012 [12, 13]. The meta-analyses included data from the INVEST, Australian, VERTOS II, and FREE trials. Overall, these revealed greater pain relief, reduced disability, and improved quality of life after vertebroplasty and kyphoplasty. For patients with neoplasm-related fractures, there are no additional randomized controlled trials, and thus no meta-analysis.

With regard to procedural safety, major complications occur in less than 1 % of patients treated for osteoporotic fractures and less than 5 % treated for neoplasm-related fractures [14]. In meta-analysis of the prospective randomized controlled trials there were no statistically significant differences in medical adverse events between vertebroplasty/kyphoplasty or conservative treatment [12]. However randomized controlled trials may be limited in the detection of rare harms. Overall, potential complications that have been reported in the literature include symptomatic extra-osseous cement leakage; radicular or spinal cord injury resulting in pain, paralysis, or bowel/bladder dysfunction; or need for emergent surgical decompression, cement or fat pulmonary emboli, osteomyelitis, rib or pedicle fracture, local vascular injury, hypotension or depressed myocardial function, pneumothorax and death from fatal cement or fat embolism, cardiovascular collapse, or cement anaphylaxis. The major source of complications is unrecognized cement leakage. The cavity created by the balloon tamp inflation during kyphoplasty does reduce the rates of overall cement leakage compared to vertebroplasty [15]; however rates of symptomatic cement leakage are similar. In addition, meta-analyses have shown that there is no increased risk of secondary vertebral fractures after vertebroplasty compared to conservative management of osteoporotic fractures [16, 17].

Patients with neoplasm-related fractures are at higher risk of complications compared to osteoporotic fractures; in particular fractures with destruction of the posterior vertebral wall or epidural tumor extension incur higher procedural risk. Importantly, patients with this fracture morphology were deemed unsuitable and hence excluded from the CAFE trial and there were no major complications. Thus both procedural effectiveness and safety have to be balanced in the treatment of individual patients.

These recent evidentiary updates have led to endorsement of vertebroplasty and kyphoplasty by the *National Institute for Health and Care Excellence (NICE)* in 2013 for patients with severe ongoing back pain from a recent vertebral fracture that is refractory to conservative medical management, if there are concordant physical examination and imaging findings. Similarly, in the last 2 years, multiple international societies have also published guidelines and position statements endorsing both vertebroplasty and kyphoplasty for selected patients who have ongoing severe pain and disability that is refractory to conservative medical management [18–20].

Implementation

Successful integration of vertebroplasty and kyphoplasty into your spine practice requires good foundational knowledge of the current evidence in the medical literature, an appropriate patient selection strategy, meticulous technique, and routine assessment of clinical outcomes.

Patient Selection

Selection of patients should focus on those who will likely benefit most from vertebroplasty and kyphoplasty. Absolute and relative contraindications are summarized in Boxes 20.1 and 20.2. Typical symptoms from a recent unhealed vertebral compression fracture include deep midline pain that is exacerbated by axial mechanical loading (typically worse with standing/weight-bearing and may be relieved by recumbency) or flexion. There may be midline or slightly off-midline tenderness at the fractured level. Localization to a particular level is especially important in patients with multiple fractures, some of which may be healed and do not require treatment. In difficult cases, physical examination can be performed with fluoroscopic assistance. If there is a clear disparity between the examination findings and imaging, or clear alternate source of back pain, vertebroplasty or kyphoplasty should not be performed.

Box 20.1 Absolute contraindications to vertebroplasty and kyphoplasty
1. Active systemic infection, in particular spinal infection.
2. Uncorrectable bleeding diathesis.
3. Insufficient cardiopulmonary health to safely tolerate sedation or general anesthesia.
4. Known anaphylaxis to bone cement.
5. Compressive myelopathy from fracture retropulsion or epidural tumoral extension.

Box 20.2 Relative contraindications to vertebroplasty and kyphoplasty
These relative contraindications substantially increase technical difficulty and risk of the procedure. Thus they should not be considered early in the integration of vertebroplasty and kyphoplasty into your spine practice.

- *Vertebroplasty above T5*. Visualization is challenging due to radiographic overlap by the shoulders. In addition, the pedicles and vertebral bodies are small.
- *Marked loss of vertebral body height* (greater than 75 % height loss). There is typically little space for cannula placement, and needle trajectories need to be extremely accurate.
- *Marked disruption of the posterior vertebral body cortex*. This increases the risk of posterior cement leakage into the spinal canal, and venous extravasation into the basivertebral vein.
- *Substantial canal narrowing*. This increases the risk that even a small amount of cement leakage could produce neurologic compromise.
- *Retropulsed fracture fragments*. If the posterior vertebral body wall is unstable, there is risk of further spinal canal compromise. Some practitioners limit treatment to patients in which retropulsion < 20 % of canal diameter [28].
- *Epidural tumoral extension*. This increases the risk of posterior cement leakage into the spinal canal.

Imaging should be performed in all cases to confirm the clinical diagnosis and assess fracture acuity. While plain radiographs are often the initial investigation, magnetic resonance imaging (MRI) is the test of choice. This should be obtained in all patients if not contraindicated. Short tau inversion recovery (STIR) or T2-weighted sequences with fat saturation are the most useful (Fig. 20.1). Unhealed fractures show hyperintense signal consistent with bone marrow edema. MRI not

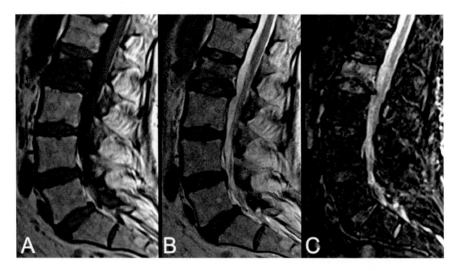

Fig. 20.1 Utility of MRI. (**a**) T1 MRI shows low attenuation in the acute L2 vertebral body fracture. (**b**) T2 MRI shows altered signal in the L2 vertebral body. (**c**) STIR MRI shows obvious increased signal in the L2 vertebral body from bone marrow edema. Use of STIR of fat-saturated T2 MRI is helpful to define the extent of bone marrow edema for appropriate patient selection. It is reasonable to exclude patients without abnormal STIR signal from treatment

only assesses fracture acuity but may also reveal other fractured levels not discernible on less sensitive modalities such as plain radiography or CT. MRI also distinguishes osteoporotic from neoplasm-related fracture, and assesses for fracture retropulsion, epidural tumor extension, spinal canal compromise, and compression of the spinal cord or nerve roots. In patients who cannot undergo MRI, nuclear scintigraphic bone scan is the test of choice. Unhealed fractures will take up the injected 99mTc-MDP tracer in much higher concentrations and this is predictive of positive clinical response after vertebral augmentation [21]. For neoplasm-related fractures, computed tomography is particularly important to assess the integrity of the posterior vertebral body cortex, which impacts on the risk of cement leakage into the spinal canal.

It is also important to document pain and disability levels using well-established scales used in the literature, such as the 10-point numeric back pain scale or visual analogue scale, and RDQ. Patients with severe ongoing back pain and disability that is refractory to conservative medical therapy should be selected for treatment. Failure of conservative therapy is variably defined, but can be considered as pain that is not adequately controlled by analgesics and/or bed rest, or intolerance to analgesics (e.g., excessive sedation from narcotic analgesia). While one should consider an initial trial of conservative therapy, there has been a growing trend to earlier treatment (within days) for highly selected patients, such as those requiring hospitalization and/or parenteral analgesia [22, 23].

Technique

The patient should be positioned prone or oblique prone for thoracic and lumbar procedures. Proper cushion support under the upper chest and lower abdomen maximizes extension promoting kyphosis reduction [24]. The patient's arms should be placed toward the head to ensure that they are not in the path of the fluoroscope. The majority of vertebroplasty and kyphoplasty can be performed with moderate conscious sedation and local analgesia; in some cases, general anesthesia is required to provide adequate comfort and safety. In all cases, continuous ECG, blood pressure, and pulse oximetry monitoring should be performed in conjunction with certified nursing personnel, nurse anesthetists, or anesthesiologists. Use standard operating-room guidelines for sterile preparation of the skin, draping, operator scrub, and sterile gowns, masks, and gloves, as well as intravenous antibiotic prophylaxis prior to skin incision.

Most often vertebroplasty and kyphoplasty are performed with fluoroscopic guidance. Have a clear understanding of the affected level and appropriate bony landmarks prior to skin incision. Use of biplane fluoroscopy reduces procedure time, and the image dose may be increased if required to help identify bony landmarks in markedly osteopenic patients. The needle may be placed via a transpedicular or parapedicular approach. The transpedicular approach passes through the posterior surface of the pedicle, via the length of the pedicle, and into the vertebral body. This long intraosseous path protects adjacent soft tissues including neural and vascular structures. However, this approach can limit the ability to achieve a midline needle tip position. The alternate parapedicular approach penetrates the pedicle along its path that permits a more central tip placement, facilitating unilateral treatment (Fig. 20.2).

The needle trajectory must be kept lateral to the medial cortex and superior to the inferior cortex of the pedicle (Fig. 20.3). This prevents entry into the spinal canal or the neural foramen. Once the needle has traversed the pedicle, it can be advanced to the anterior aspect of the vertebral body. If a curved vertebroplasty needle is used, different areas of the vertebral body can be targeted (Fig. 20.4). Once in position the needle stylet is removed, and the cannula filled with saline to prevent pressurized injection of air and secondary embolus. Subsequently, cement can be injected through the percutaneous cannula into the bone. For kyphoplasty, after initial positioning the cannula is pulled back slightly into the posterior aspect of the vertebral body to create room to allow for the insertion and inflation of a balloon tamp. The tamp creates a cavity into which cement is injected (Fig. 20.5). The long flexible cement delivery systems minimize radiation exposure to the operator [25]. Careful fluoroscopic monitoring is performed during cement injection. Any extraosseous cement extravasation should be avoided; in particular posterior or posterolateral leakage could result in irritation or injury to the spinal cord or nerve roots. The optimal volume of cement remains a matter of controversy. Small volumes of cement continue to result in good clinical outcomes after vertebroplasty [26]. Attempting to place a large volume of cement may in turn lead to higher rates of

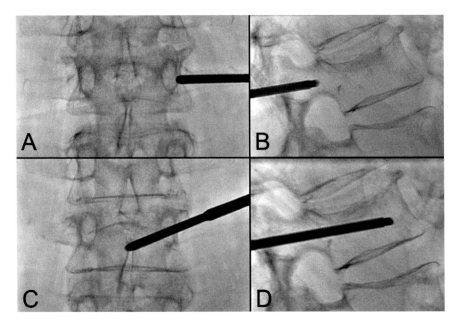

Fig. 20.2 Unilateral parapedicular approach. (**a**) AP fluoroscopic image shows the needle tip entry position at the lateral margin of the pedicle. (**b**) Lateral fluoroscopic image shows needle tip entry position halfway along the pedicle. AP (**c**) and lateral (**d**) fluoroscopic images demonstrating final midline needle tip position achieved in the anterior third of the vertebral body

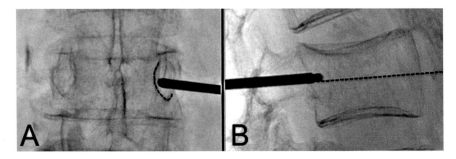

Fig. 20.3 Importance of the medial and inferior pedicle cortices. (**a**) AP fluoroscopic image. During the entire course of transpedicular needle access, the medial and inferior pedicle cortices must remain visible until the entire pedicle has been traversed on the lateral projection (**b**). Note that the entire needle trajectory within the vertebral body should be considered during initial transpedicular access for optimal final needle position

extra-osseous leakage and symptomatic complications; similarly cement fill in the posterior third of the vertebral body close to the basivertebral vein is best avoided. The needle may be reinserted to deliver the final portion of cement, and after allowing the cement to harden, the needle and cannula are removed with a gentle rocking motion to prevent cement migrating along the needle tract.

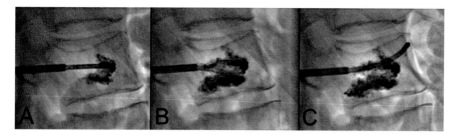

Fig. 20.4 Utility of the curved vertebroplasty needle. (**a**) Lateral fluoroscopic image demonstrating the curved needle tip with cement injection in a pathological L1 fracture. (**b**) Lateral fluoroscopic images with the curved needle repositioned to a target inferior bony compartment. (**c**) Lateral fluoroscopic images with the curved needle repositioned to a target superior bony compartment

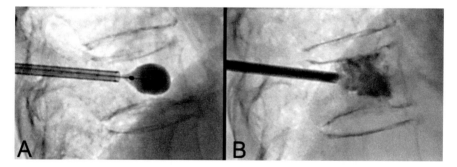

Fig. 20.5 Unilateral balloon kyphoplasty. (**a**) Lateral fluoroscopic image shows the balloon tamp inflated within the vertebral body. (**b**) Lateral fluoroscopic image shows the cement infected into the balloon cavity and adjacent trabecular bone. Note that the cement fill has been limited to the anterior two-thirds of the vertebral body to avoid basivertebral venous extravasation

Post-procedure Care and Clinical Outcomes

Afterward, the patient should have a period of observation of vital signs and lower limb neurological function as well as bed rest (for example 2 h). This also allows the cement to fully harden and integrate before axial load of the spine. Most patients can be discharged later on the same day. Any clinical deterioration suspicious for local cement leakage should prompt cross-sectional imaging with CT and/or MRI. Systemic or cardiorespiratory deterioration is suspicious for cement or fat pulmonary embolism, and should prompt chest imaging.

Post-procedure follow-up should reassess previously recorded pain and disability scale scores. These procedures should be performed within a quality improvement program where the clinical effectiveness and safety can be examined. Rates of all major permanent complications should be <2 %, including in neoplasm-related fractures [27]. Greater than 1 % permanent neurological deficit rate for osteoporotic fractures and 5 % for neoplasm-related fractures should prompt additional review of practice [27].

Summary

Successful integration of vertebroplasty and kyphoplasty into your spine practice requires a good understanding of the evidence in the medical literature, appropriate patient selection, meticulous technique, and routine assessment of clinical outcomes. There is sufficient data to support the use of vertebroplasty and kyphoplasty in selected patients with osteoporotic or neoplasm-related vertebral fracture-related pain and disability that is refractory to conservative therapy. All published trials have limitations, and further trials are ongoing. In the meantime, practitioners who perform these procedures should use strict patient selection and meticulous technique to maximize the excellent safety profile and monitor their clinical effectiveness, ideally within the setting of a quality improvement program.

References

1. Cooper C, O'Neill T, Silman A. The epidemiology of vertebral fractures. European Vertebral Osteoporosis Study Group. Bone. 1993;14 Suppl 1:S89–97.
2. Kawaguchi S, Horigome K, Yajima H, et al. Symptomatic relevance of intravertebral cleft in patients with osteoporotic vertebral fracture. J Neurosurg Spine. 2010;13(2):267–75.
3. Hussein MA, Vrionis FD, Allison R, et al. The role of vertebral augmentation in multiple myeloma: International Myeloma Working Group Consensus Statement. Leukemia. 2008;22(8):1479–84.
4. Boehling NS, Grosshans DR, Allen PK, et al. Vertebral compression fracture risk after stereotactic body radiotherapy for spinal metastases. J Neurosurg Spine. 2012;16(4):379–86.
5. Cunha MV, Al-Omair A, Atenafu EG, et al. Vertebral compression fracture (VCF) after spine stereotactic body radiation therapy (SBRT): analysis of predictive factors. Int J Radiat Oncol Biol Phys. 2012;84(3):e343–9.
6. Rose PS, Laufer I, Boland PJ, et al. Risk of fracture after single fraction image-guided intensity-modulated radiation therapy to spinal metastases. J Clin Oncol. 2009;27(30):5075–9.
7. Kallmes DF, Comstock BA, Heagerty PJ, et al. A randomized trial of vertebroplasty for osteoporotic spinal fractures. N Engl J Med. 2009;361(6):569–79.
8. Buchbinder R, Osborne RH, Ebeling PR, et al. A randomized trial of vertebroplasty for painful osteoporotic vertebral fractures. N Engl J Med. 2009;361(6):557–68.
9. Wardlaw D, Cummings SR, Van Meirhaeghe J, et al. Efficacy and safety of balloon kyphoplasty compared with non-surgical care for vertebral compression fracture (FREE): a randomised controlled trial. Lancet. 2009;373(9668):1016–24.
10. Klazen CA, Lohle PN, de Vries J, et al. Vertebroplasty versus conservative treatment in acute osteoporotic vertebral compression fractures (Vertos II): an open-label randomised trial. Lancet. 2010;376(9746):1085–92.
11. Berenson J, Pflugmacher R, Jarzem P, et al. Balloon kyphoplasty versus non-surgical fracture management for treatment of painful vertebral body compression fractures in patients with cancer: a multicentre, randomised controlled trial. Lancet Oncol. 2011;12(3):225–35.
12. Anderson PA, Froyshteter AB, Tontz Jr WL. Meta-analysis of vertebral augmentation compared to conservative treatment for osteoporotic spinal fractures. J Bone Miner Res. 2013;28:372–82.
13. Shi MM, Cai XZ, Lin T, et al. Is there really no benefit of vertebroplasty for osteoporotic vertebral fractures? A meta-analysis. Clin Orthop Relat Res. 2012;470(10):2785–99.

14. McGraw JK, Cardella J, Barr JD, et al. Society of Interventional Radiology quality improvement guidelines for percutaneous vertebroplasty. J Vasc Interv Radiol. 2003;14(9 Pt 2):S311–5.
15. Xiao H, Yang J, Feng X, et al. Comparing complications of vertebroplasty and kyphoplasty for treating osteoporotic vertebral compression fractures: a meta-analysis of the randomized and non-randomized controlled studies. Eur J Orthop Surg Traumatol. 2015;25:S77–85.
16. Han SL, Wan SL, Li QT, et al. Is vertebroplasty a risk factor for subsequent vertebral fracture, meta-analysis of published evidence? Osteoporos Int. 2015;26(1):113–22.
17. Song D, Meng B, Gan M, et al. The incidence of secondary vertebral fracture of vertebral augmentation techniques versus conservative treatment for painful osteoporotic vertebral fractures: a systematic review and meta-analysis. Acta Radiol. 2015;56:970–9.
18. Barr JD, Jensen ME, Hirsch JA, et al. Position statement on percutaneous vertebral augmentation: a consensus statement developed by the Society of Interventional Radiology (SIR), American Association of Neurological Surgeons (AANS) and the Congress of Neurological Surgeons (CNS), American College of Radiology (ACR), American Society of Neuroradiology (ASNR), American Society of Spine Radiology (ASSR), Canadian Interventional Radiology Association (CIRA), and the Society of NeuroInterventional Surgery (SNIS). J Vasc Interv Radiol. 2014;25(2):171–81.
19. Chandra RV, Meyers PM, Hirsch JA, et al. Vertebral augmentation: report of the Standards and Guidelines Committee of the Society of NeuroInterventional Surgery. J Neurointerv Surg. 2014;6(1):7–15.
20. Terpos E, Morgan G, Dimopoulos MA, et al. International Myeloma Working Group recommendations for the treatment of multiple myeloma-related bone disease. J Clin Oncol. 2013;31(18):2347–57.
21. Maynard AS, Jensen ME, Schweickert PA, et al. Value of bone scan imaging in predicting pain relief from percutaneous vertebroplasty in osteoporotic vertebral fractures. AJNR Am J Neuroradiol. 2000;21(10):1807–12.
22. Stallmeyer MJB, Zoarski GH, Obuchowski AM. Optimizing patient selection in percutaneous vertebroplasty. J Vasc Interv Radiol. 2003;14(6):683–96.
23. Kallmes DF, Jensen ME. Percutaneous vertebroplasty. Radiology. 2003;229(1):27–36. doi:10.1148/radiol.2291020222 [published Online First: Epub Date].
24. Teng MM, Wei CJ, Wei LC, et al. Kyphosis correction and height restoration effects of percutaneous vertebroplasty. AJNR Am J Neuroradiol. 2003;24(9):1893–900.
25. Komemushi A, Tanigawa N, Kariya S, et al. Radiation exposure to operators during vertebroplasty. J Vasc Interv Radiol. 2005;16(10):1327–32.
26. Kaufmann TJ, Trout AT, Kallmes DF. The effects of cement volume on clinical outcomes of percutaneous vertebroplasty. AJNR Am J Neuroradiol. 2006;27(9):1933–7.
27. Baerlocher MO, Saad WE, Dariushnia S, et al. Quality improvement guidelines for percutaneous vertebroplasty. J Vasc Interv Radiol. 2014;25(2):165–70.
28. Jensen ME, Dion JE. Percutaneous vertebroplasty in the treatment of osteoporotic compression fractures. Neuroimaging Clin N Am. 2000;10(3):547–68.

Chapter 21
Emerging Technology in Neuromodulation: Waveforms and New Targets in Spinal Cord Stimulation

Timothy R. Deer and Chong H. Kim

Key Points

- Conventional spinal cord stimulation (SCS) requires perceived therapeutic paresthesia overlapping the patient's pain mapping area.
- Conventional SCS systems typically use a frequency between 40 and 100 Hz.
- In conventional SCS, leads are commonly placed midline or slightly off midline in the posterior epidural space to stimulate the dorsal columns.
- Challenges exist with conventional SCS, including unpleasant and unwanted paresthesias, postural stimulation changes, and the inability to cover discrete regions of the body.
- Burst stimulation delivers 40 Hz bursts with 5 spikes at 500 Hz per burst with a specific waveform construct.
- High-frequency (HF10) stimulation waveforms at 10,000 Hz with a specific shape and characteristic.
- In initial prospective and observational publications, burst, and HF10 modalities have been shown to improve outcomes in patients that have failed conventional frequency tonic SCS.
- Both HF10 and burst stimulation achieve pain treatment without the need to achieve paresthesia. HF10 is paresthesia free and burst is sub-threshold.
- Paresthesia-free stimulation may change the pain care algorithm for both axial back pain with or without radicular complaints. Initial data is very encouraging from both the USA and international data.

T.R. Deer, M.D. (✉)
Center for Pain Relief, Inc., 400 Court St., Suite 100, Charleston, WV 25301, USA
e-mail: doctdeer@aol.com

C.H. Kim, M.D.
Neurosurgery, Division of Pain Management, Health Sciences Center, West Virginia University, Suite 4300, PO Box 9183, Morgantown, WV 26506, USA
e-mail: kimc@wvuhealthcare.com

© Springer International Publishing Switzerland 2016
S.M. Falowski, J.E. Pope (eds.), *Integrating Pain Treatment into Your Spine Practice*, DOI 10.1007/978-3-319-27796-7_21

- Dorsal root ganglion (DRG) stimulation may provide more selective and consistent targeting of painful areas than conventional SCS. DRG stimulation, in initial studies, has produced discrete prescribed paresthesia that is specific to the areas of abnormal nerve function.
- DRG stimulation has been able to achieve pain relief at a sub-threshold or paresthesia-free level of energy in early reports from Australia and Europe.

Introduction

Spinal cord stimulation (SCS) is a commonly accepted treatment option for neuropathic pain [1–4]. Despite the growing evidence of clinical efficacy, there are a number of patients that fail this therapy because of unwanted paresthesia, failure to cover an area of painful neural stimulus, excessive energy requirements, or lack of pain relief. Conventional SCS uses a fixed pulse width and amplitude and low frequency to replace the painful sensation with a better tolerated sensation, also known as paresthesia. Additionally, in conventional SCS, the leads are placed in the posterior epidural space, most commonly on or near midline, to stimulate the dorsal column. Ideally, the paresthesia should only be localized to the areas of pain, without stimulation of unwanted areas, and the paresthesia should be pleasant, without variations regardless of movement or postural change [5–8]. Considering that it is easier to stimulate a normal nerve than an abnormal nerve in the dorsal column, it is not surprising that patients often fail this therapy when they have specific pain such as the foot or groin. Unfortunately in the use of conventional SCS, failure in any of these aspects can lead to the failure of SCS treatment.

Advances are under way with new technologies, new strategies in electrical waveform delivery, frequency, and targets for stimulation to address these areas of concern and to improve the outcome in the use of SCS.

Evidence

The most accepted mechanistic proposal for the action of SCS is based on the gate control theory proposed by Melzack and Wall, that activity in large-diameter cutaneous fibers (type Aß) inhibits the transmission of noxious information to the brain by small (C and Ad) fibers. Therefore, it has been postulated that electrical stimulation could activate these large fibers and that this would ultimately suppress pain transmitting small secondary neurons [9]. Conventional treatment of neuropathic and chronic pain with SCS is based on tonic stimulation, with the pain relief dependent on perceived therapeutic paresthesia coverage of the typical areas of pain. The described mechanism of conventional SCS in pain relief is likely related to a combination of a spinal and supraspinal mechanisms [10, 11]. This includes antidromic activation of ascending dorsal column fibers and orthodromic activation of

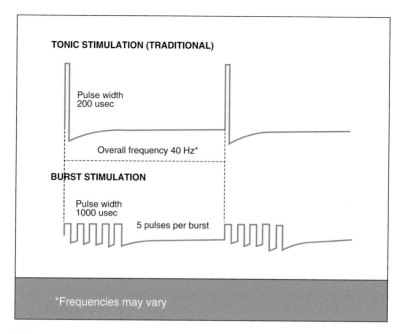

Fig. 21.1 Comparison of traditional and burst stimulation waveforms. Courtesy of St. Jude Medical

ascending fibers with descending serotoninergic pain modulatory systems [12–15]. New advances in waveform and frequency challenge the traditional paradigm with pain relief without perceived paresthesia. Conventional SCS uses tonic stimulation, performed using either a constant current or a constant voltage generator that induces electrical signals at the level of the spinal cord. Tonic stimulation describes the waveform characteristics of the energy applied, typically a continuous frequency, regardless of the type of system power source (constant current or voltage). Conventional SCS applies stimulation frequencies most commonly between 40 and 100 Hz. In contrast, high-frequency (HF10) and burst stimulation delivers the energy at much higher frequencies and at very-well-defined waveform morphology. HF10 stimulation provides a unique waveform with fixed pulse width and frequency delivered at 10,000 Hz while burst stimulation delivers groups of pulses at 500 Hz in a specific waveform fingerprint [16–18].

Burst SCS uses small bursts of pulses of stimulation, rather than the continuous pulses to provide pain relief, without eliciting paresthesia [17]. Burst programing delivers groups of pulses, called burst trains separated by quiescent periods. Each burst train contains a series of pulses at constant pulse amplitude, pulse width, and interpulse frequency (Fig. 21.1). Burst stimulation is based on the ability to emit significantly more energy per second than traditional tonic stimulation. As a result, lower temporal integration is considered to be required to reach the excitation threshold of a neuron, thereby activating neurons that cannot be influenced by tonic stimulation [17, 19]. This stimulation below the threshold for activation of the Aß fibers is believed to result in the paresthesia-free pain relief. Burst stimulation is based on the knowledge of dual-firing properties of thalamic cells, including tonic and burst modes [20]. Thalamic burst stimulation can activate the cortex more effectively than tonic firing [15]. This eventually led to research of its activity on the spinal cord [17]. Burst stimulation consists of intermittent packets of closely spaced, high-frequency stimuli with five spikes at 500 Hz per burst, with a pulse width of 1 millisecond (ms) and 1 ms interspike interval delivered in constant current mode. The cumulative charge of the five 1 ms spikes is balanced during 5 ms after the spikes, which differentiates it from high-frequency clustered firing, in which each pulse is immediately charge balanced [18]. It is hypothesized that the affective component of pain is separate, and distinctly different than the perceptive pathway. It is theorized, and evidence suggests, that burst stimulation works by modulating both the medial (affective) and lateral (perceptive) [17, 18].

Burst stimulation has been studied extensively. In a double-blind placebo-controlled trial comparing tonic stimulation with burst stimulation with placebo, burst stimulation statistically significantly improved pain reduction for general pain, back pain, and leg pain [19]. Additionally, at clinically useful amplitudes, burst stimulation waveform provided analgesia without a reliance on perceived paresthesia [18]. In another study, patients that had traditional, tonic stimulation for at least 6 months were given burst stimulation for 2 weeks. The patients were grouped into three categories: diabetic peripheral neuropathy (DPN), failed back surgery syndrome (FBSS), and FBSS-poor responders (FBSS-PR). FBSS-PR was defined as patients with failed back surgery syndrome plus poor or lost therapeutic benefit from their SCS device. Interestingly, the visual analog scale (VAS) was reduced nearly 62 % on average with burst-SCS compared to 37 % with SCS. Additionally, the effect compared to tonic stimulation was largest for PDN (decreased 77 %), as compared to FBSS (decreased 57 %), or FBSS-PR (23 %) [21]. Another study similarly examined previously SCS-implanted patients and intervened with 2 weeks of burst stimulation [22]. VAS reduced 46 % with the burst stimulation with 73 % of the patients reporting no paresthesia while 23 % reported a reduction. Overall, 91 % preferred the burst stimulation. A prospective, randomized, double-blinded, placebo-controlled study examined the burst stimulation to 500 Hz tonic stimulation and to placebo stimulation in FBSS subjects [23]. Overall, burst stimulation resulted in significantly better pain relief and improved pain quality. It is important to note that since burst stimulation has energy requirements that are usually less than traditional tonic stimulation, primary or rechargeable battery can be used.

No complications were reported to be associated strictly with burst-SCS. Recently, a randomized multicenter comparative efficacy study evaluating burst to tonic stimulation has been fully enrolled in the USA under FDA pivotal monitoring (Sunburst, St. Jude Neuro division, Plano, Texas). The results of this study, which has a non-inferiority design, should be available by the fall of 2015.

HF10 therapy is another advance heralded as providing analgesia without paresthesia. HF10 (Nevro, Menlo Park) is capable of delivering frequencies from 2 to 10,000 Hz but the therapy is always delivered at 10,000 Hz compared to the 40 to 100 Hz typically used in conventional SCS. At this time, it is the only FDA-approved

Waveform Comparison

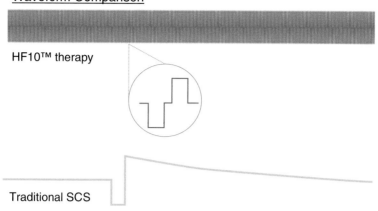

HF10™ therapy

Traditional SCS

Fig. 21.2 Comparison of traditional and HF10™ therapy waveforms. Courtesy of Nevro Corp

paresthesia-free therapy. HF10 therapy uses biphasic charge-balanced pulse train with pulse widths usually set to 30 microsecond and a uniform frequency (Fig. 21.2). Like all forms of SCS it has been theorized that HF10 therapy may also impact both spinal and supraspinal mechanism pathways, but the mechanism of action is not currently fully elucidated. Preclinical work in animal models suggests the ability of HF10 SCS to suppress hypersensitized wide dynamic range cells [24].

Several studies have shown HF10 to be efficacious in treatment of chronic pain. One studied predominant back pain patients, who were trialed sequentially with traditional SCS and then HF-10 SCS [16]. At the end of the sequential trials, HF10 stimulation reduced VAS 77 % from baseline, with a responder rate of 83 %, while traditional SCS had a VAS reduction from baseline of 55 %, with a 58 % responder rate. 88 % preferred HF10 over traditional SCS. Although HF10 performed better than traditional SCS, both methods significantly produced a reduction in baseline pain. A European multicenter trial yielded similar findings [25, 26]. Patients were implanted with HF10 SCS and followed for 6 months [25]. 88 % of the patients trialed with HF10 were converted to the permanent therapy. At 6 months, the average baseline back pain VAS was improved to 2.4 from 8.4. The ODI at 6 months improved to 37 from 55. Of note, 74 % of the patients at 6 months were defined as responders (having a greater than 50 % VAS improvement in their pain) and 85 % of the patients reported satisfaction with HF10. This study also showed improvement in the use of opioids. Of the 86 % of the patients who were using opioids at baseline, 38 % eliminated their need for opioids and 62 % reduced them. At 24 months, average VAS back pain was 3.3 from 8.4 and leg pain 2.3 from 5.4 [26]. Finally, a multicenter, prospective, randomized, controlled trial (SENZA-RCT) showed that 84.5 % of implanted HF10 therapy subjects were responders for back pain and 83.1 % for leg pain. In comparison, in the controlled group consisting of traditional SCS subjects, 43.8 % were responders for back pain and 55.5 % for leg pain. The superiority of the paresthesia-free HF10 group continued to show superiority at 12 months [27].

In a study in Switzerland, investigators studied stimulation at 5 kHz to sham (no stimulation) and tonic stimulation in a double-blind, two period crossover, randomized control trial [28]. They reported that only 14/33 patients responded to the 5 kHz stimulation, and the 5 kHz stimulation was equivalent to sham for primary outcome measures. This may suggest that the results are inherently dependent on the frequency used for stimulation, and not all high-frequency stimulation is equal. The study had many questions on method however such as lead placement, preconditioning to tonic stimulation, and patient selection that many feel no valid conclusions can be made. HF10 stimulation requires a much higher energy burden as compared to conventional or burst stimulation. There is no evidence that this may impact battery life but daily charging is required. With the constraints of current battery technology, HF10 stimulation at this time is used with rechargeable technology. Since the HF10 SCS stimulation does not require a paresthesia for analgesia, and based on years of empirical work programming patients, the area of stimulation for this therapy is between T8 and T11, and the leads can be placed with the implant procedure performed with the patients in continual sedation with placement based on anatomical landmarks in the midline.

The complication rate of the HF10 appears to be the same as compared to traditional SCS, and there is no evidence in the human or animal that higher frequencies cause neural damage.

Dorsal root ganglion (DRG) stimulation involves placement of a novel electrode lead on the surface of the DRG. The DRG contains cell bodies of primary sensory neurons. There are several types of DRG neurons and they are known to participate in the signaling process as well as modulation of this process [29]. This includes sensory processing of nociceptive pain and the development of neuropathic pain. As a result, the DRG has long been a clinical target for pain control, most recently with neuromodulation [30–39]. The location of the DRG is consistent and is always in the epidural space between the medial and lateral aspects of the pedicle with the neural foramen and is made up of the dorsal sensory root fiber cell bodies as dorsal afferent sensory axons and ventral efferent motor axons form the respective rootlets. The DRG is accessed for neurostimulation from an epidural approach using a DRG lead-specific sheath (Fig. 21.3). The DRG lead is much smaller than conventional leads and has a unique shape. It is theorized that electrical stimulation around the DRG may decrease hyperexcitability of the DRG neurons and thereby provide relief of chronic aberrant pain.

DRG stimulation was initially studied in a prospective, single-arm, pilot study [37]. The results showed 70 % overall reduction in pain as well as reduction in pain medication use. Pain relief in the foot was even more vigorous at over 80 %, which is encouraging considering that this can be a difficult target with conventional dorsal column stimulation. A larger multicenter prospective trial studied DRG stimulation in chronic pain of limb and/or trunk [38]. At 6 months, average overall pain ratings were 58 % lower than baseline, with more than half the subjects reporting greater than 50 % relief. The proportions of subjects experiencing 50 % or more reduction in pain specific to back, leg, and foot regions were 57 %, 70 %, and 89 %, respectively. The study had two reversal periods in which the stimulation was turned off, during which time, the pain returned to baseline levels. Furthermore, the results

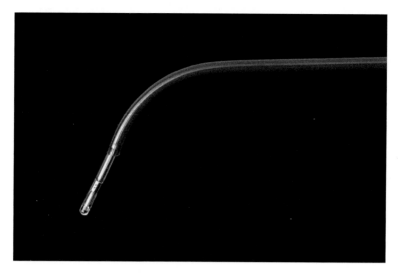

Fig. 21.3 Image of DRG lead sheath. Courtesy of St. Jude Medical/Spinal Modulation Inc

showed stable paresthesia intensity over time with no significant difference in the paresthesia intensity perceived during different body postures/positions (standing up vs. lying down). The subjects continued to experience benefit at 12 months [40]. Pain was reduced by 56 % at 12 months post-implantation, and 60 % of subjects reported greater than 50 % improvement in their pain with DRG stimulation. Pain localized to the back, legs, and feet was reduced by 42 %, 62 %, and 80 %, respectively.

In addition to pain improvement and stable paresthesia intensities independent of body position, DRG stimulation may be better able to capture discrete painful areas such as the feet or groin [41, 42]. DRG stimulation modality may allow for more selective and consistent targeting of painful areas than conventional SCS.

DRG stimulation has been attempted with conventional SCS systems; however currently approved systems are large and may compress the DRG within the foramen. Additionally, the size and spacing of the electrodes are not designed to target the DRG and may recruit and stimulate other structures. The new system is specifically designed to address these issues, to safely, comfortably, and optimally stimulate the DRG.

In the 12-month prospective study, the most common adverse events were temporary motor stimulation, cerebral spinal fluid leak with associated headaches, and infection. The two most frequent adverse events were attributed to implant procedure and programming of the novice device and technique. The infection rates were comparable to conventional published rates.

Recently, the results of the US pivotal study on DRG stimulation as compared to conventional stimulation were presented at the International Neuromodulation Society meeting [43]. In this FDA-monitored study, DRG showed both non-inferiority and superiority as compared to conventional spinal cord stimulation in the treatment of neuropathic pain of the groin and lower limb [44].

Implementation

Advances in waveform with burst stimulation, high-frequency stimulation with HF-10 and new target with DRG stimulation offer new ways and target to deliver energy. These appear to offer advantages over conventional spinal cord tonic stimulation. HF10 and burst stimulation may offer advantages over tonic stimulation including better patient tolerance with paresthesia-free stimulation, comparable increase in function, and possible success with a subset of patient population refractory to conventional or tonic spinal cord stimulation. In addition to pain improvement and stable paresthesia intensities independent of body position, DRG stimulation may allow more selective targeting of painful areas. These new advances may improve the trial to permanent conversions and more importantly improve therapy sustainability.

Summary

Advances are under way in electrical waveform delivery, frequency, and targets for stimulation to address the concerns of conventional SCS and more importantly to improve the outcome in the use of SCS. This is truly an era of innovation that may revolutionize the field and improve patient care and outcomes.

References

1. Kumar K, Taylor RS, Jacques L, et al. Spinal cord stimulation versus conventional medical management for neuropathic pain: a multicentre randomized controlled trial in patients with failed back surgery syndrome. Pain. 2007;132:179–88.
2. Kumar K, Taylor RS, Jacques L, et al. The effects of spinal cord stimulation in neuropathic pain are sustained: a 24-month follow-up of the prospective randomized controlled multicenter trial of effectiveness of spinal cord stimulation. Neurosurgery. 2008;63:762–70.
3. North RB, Kidd DH, Farrokhi F, Piantadosi SA. Spinal cord stimulation versus repeated lumbosacral spine surgery for chronic pain: a randomized controlled trial. Neurosurgery. 2005;56:98–106.
4. Taylor RS, Van Buyten JP, Buschser E. Spinal cord stimulation for complex regional pain syndrome: a systematic review of the clinical and cost-effectiveness literature and assessment of prognostic factors. Eur J Pain. 2006;10:91–101.
5. De Leon-Casasola OA. Spinal cord and peripheral nerve stimulation techniques for neuropathic pain. J Pain Symptom Manage. 2009;38:S28–38.
6. North RB, Ewend MG, Lawton MT, Piantadosi SA. Spinal cord stimulation for chronic, intractable pain: superiority of "multi-channel" devices. Pain. 1991;44:119–30.
7. Frey ME, Manchikanti L, Benyamin RM, et al. Spinal cord stimulation for patients with failed back surgery syndrome: a systematic review. Pain Physician. 2009;12:379–97.
8. Kuechmann C, Valine T, Wolfe DL. 853 Could automatic position adaptive stimulation be useful in spinal cord stimulation? Eur J Pain. 2009;113:S243c–S243.
9. Melzack R, Wall PD. Pain mechanisms: a new theory. Science. 1965;150:971–9.

10. Barchini J, Tchachaghian S, Shamaa F, Jabbur SJ, Meyerson BA, Song Z, Linderoth B, Saade NE. Spinal segmental and supraspinal mechanisms underlying the pain-relieving effects of spinal cord stimulation: an experimental study in a rat model of neuropathy. Neuroscience. 2012;215:196–208.

11. Tiede J, Brown L, Gekht G, Vallejo R, Yearwood T, Morgan D. Novel spinal cord stimulation parameters in patients with predominant back pain. Neuromodulation. 2013;16(4):370–5.

12. Saade NE, Jabbur SJ. Nociceptive behavior in animal models for peripheral neuropathy: spinal and supraspinal mechanisms. Prog Neurobiol. 2008;86:22–47.

13. De Ridder D, Vanneste S, Plaizer M, van der Loo E, Menovsky T. Burst spinal cord stimulation: toward paresthesia-free pain suppression. Neurosurgery. 2010;66(5):986–90.

14. Song Z, Ultenius C, Meyerson BA, Linderoth B. Pain relief by spinal cord stimulation involves serotonergic mechanisms: an experimental study in a rat model of mononeuropathy. Pain. 2009;147:241–8.

15. De Ridder D, Plaizer M, Kamerling N, Menovsky T, Vanneste S. Burst spinal cord stimulation for limb and back pain. World Neurosurg. 2013;80(5):642–9.

16. North RB, Roark GL. Spinal cord stimulation for chronic pain. Neurosurg Clin N Am. 1995;6:145–55.

17. Ochoa JL, Torebjork HE. Paraesthesiae from ectopic impulse generation in human sensory nerves. Brain. 1980;103:835–53, 198.

18. Meyerson BA, Linderoth B. Mode of action of spinal cord stimulation in neuropathic pain. J Pain Symptom Manage. 2006;31:S6–12.

19. Moller A. Neural plasticity and disorders of the nervous system. Cambridge, UK: Cambridge University Press; 2006.

20. Jahnsen H, Llinas R. Voltage-dependent burst-to-tonic switching of thalamic cell activity: an in vitro study. Arch Ital Biol. 1984;122:73–82.

21. De Vos CC, Bom MJ, Vanneste S, Lenders M, de Ridder D. Burst spinal cord stimulation evaluated in patients with failed back surgery syndrome and painful diabetic neuropathy. Neuromodulation. 2014;17(2):152–9.

22. Courtney P, Espinet A, Mitchell B, Russo M, Muir A, Verrills P, Davis K. Improved pain relief with burst spinal cord stimulation for two weeks in patients using tonic stimulation: results from a small clinical study. Neuromodulation. 2015. doi:10.1111/ner.12294 [Epub ahead of print].

23. Schu S, Slotty PJ, Bara G, von Knop M, Edgar D, Vespar J. A prospective, double-blinded, placebo-controlled study to examine the effectiveness of burst spinal cord stimulation patterns for the treatment of failed back surgery syndrome. Neuromodulation. 2014;17:442–50.

24. Cuellar JM, Alataris K, Walker A, Yeomans DC, Antognini JF. Effect of high-frequency alternating current on spinal afferent nociceptive transmission. Neuromodulation. 2012. doi:10.1111/ner.12015 [Epub ahead of print].

25. Van Buyten JP, Al-Kaisy A, Smet I, Palmisani S, Smith T. High frequency spinal cord stimulation of the treatment of chronic back pain patients: results of a prospective multicenter European clinical study. Neuromodulation. 2013;16(1):59–65.

26. Al-Kaisy A, Van Buyten JP, Smet I, Palmisani S, Pang D, Smith T. Sustained effectiveness of 10 kHz high frequency spinal cord stimulation for patients with chronic, low back pain: 24-month results of a prospective multicenter study. Pain Med. 2014;15(3):347–54.

27. Kapural L, Yu C, Doust M, Gliner BE, Vallejo R, Sitzman T, et al. Novel 10-kHz high-frequency therapy (HF10 therapy) is superior to traditional low-frequency spinal cord stimulation for the treatment of chronic back and leg pain: the SENZA-RCT randomized controlled trial. Anesthesiology. 2015. doi:10.1097/ALN.0000000000000774.

28. Perruchound C, Eldabe S, Batterham AM, Madzinga G, et al. Analgesia efficacy of high frequency spinal cord stimulation: a randomized, double blind placebo controlled study. Neuromodulation. 2013;16(4):363–9.

29. Devor M. Unexplained peculiarities of the dorsal root ganglion. Pain. 1999;6:S27–35.

30. Manchikanti L. Transforaminal lumbar epidural steroid injections. Pain Physician. 2000;3:374–98.

31. Vad VB, Bhat AL, Lutz GE, Cammisa F. Transforaminal epidural steroid injections in lumbosacral radiculopathy: a prospective randomized study. Spine. 2002;27:11–5.
32. Acar F, Miller J, Golshani KJ, et al. Pain relief after cervical ganglionectomy (C2 and C3) for the treatment of medically intractable occipital neuralgia. Stereotact Funct Neurosurg. 2008;86:106–12.
33. Nash TP. Percutaneous radiofrequency lesioning of dorsal root ganglia for intractable pain. Pain. 1986;24:67–73.
34. Lord SM, Barnsley L, Wallis BJ, et al. Percutaneous radio-frequency neurotomy for chronic cervical zygapophyseal joint pain. N Engl J Med. 1996;335:1721–6.
35. DeLouw AJA, Vles HSH, Freling G, et al. The morphological effects of a radio frequency lesion adjacent to the dorsal root ganglion (RF-DRG): an experimental study in the goat. Eur J Pain. 2001;5:169–74.
36. Van Zundert J, Patijn J, Kessels A, et al. Pulsed radiofrequency adjacent to the cervical dorsal root ganglion in chronic cervical radicular pain: a double blind sham controlled randomized clinical trial. Pain. 2007;127:173–82.
37. Deer TR, Grigsby E, Weiner RL, Wilcosky B, Kramer JM. A prospective study of dorsal root ganglion stimulation for the relief of chronic pain. Neuromodulation. 2013;16:67–72.
38. Liem L, Russo M, Huygen FJ, et al. A multicenter, prospective trial to assess the safety and performance of the spinal modulation dorsal root ganglion neurostimulator system in the treatment of chronic pain. Neuromodulation. 2013;16:471–82.
39. Pope JE, Deer TR, Kramer J. A systematic review: current and future directions of dorsal root ganglion therapeutics to treat chronic pain. Pain Med. 2013;14:1477–96.
40. Liem L, Russo M, Huygen FJ, et al. One-year outcomes of spinal cord stimulation of the dorsal root ganglion in the treatment of chronic neuropathic pain. Neuromodulation. 2015;18:41–9.
41. Van Buyten JP, Smet I, Liem L, Russo M, Huygen F. Stimulation of dorsal root ganglia for the management of complex regional pain syndrome: a prospective case series. Pain Pract. 2015;15:208–16.
42. Schu S, Gulve A, ElDabe S, Baranidharan G, Wolf K, Demmel W, Rasche D, Sharma M, Klase D, Jahnichen G, Wahlstedt A, Nijhuis H, Liem L. Spinal cord stimulation of the dorsal root ganglion for groin pain—a retrospective review. Pain Pract. 2015;15:293–9.
43. Deer T, Levy R. Results of the U.S. pivotal study. Montreal, Quebec, Canada. 2015.
44. Available at http://clinicaltrials.gov/ct2/show/NCT01923285, Accessed June 25 2015.

Index

© Springer International Publishing Switzerland 2016
S.M. Falowski, J.E. Pope (eds.), *Integrating Pain Treatment into Your Spine
Practice*, DOI 10.1007/978-3-319-27796-7

Printed in the United States
By Bookmasters